# ELEMENTARY
# HEARING SCIENCE

# ELEMENTARY HEARING SCIENCE

by
Lawrence J. Deutsch, Ph.D.
*Queens College of the City University of New York*
and
Alan M. Richards, Ph.D.
*Lehman College of the City University of New York*

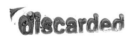

University Park Press
*Baltimore*

**UNIVERSITY PARK PRESS**
International Publishers in Science, Medicine, and Education
233 East Redwood Street
Baltimore, Maryland 21202

Typeset by American Graphic Arts Corporation
Manufactured in the United States of America by The Maple Press Company

**Library of Congress Cataloging in Publication Data**
Deutsch, Lawrence J
Elementary hearing science.

Bibliography: p.
1. Hearing.   I. Richards, Alan M., joint author.
II. Title.   [DNLM: 1. Hearing.   WV270.3 D486e]
QP461.D46        612'.85        79-419
ISBN 0-8391-1255-6

OCT 3 '79

# Contents

# Preface

This book is designed to be an introductory text in hearing and hearing loss for beginning students in audiology, speech pathology, and psychology, and a basic reference for otologists, pediatricians, and other physicians, as well as hearing aid dispensers and nurses.

As we wrote *Elementary Hearing Science*, we always kept the subtitle "What every clinician should know about hearing science" in the back of our minds. Our goal was to write a basic text for the undergraduate and beginning graduate student that introduced the major areas in the field, yet was not overwhelming in detail.

We were, of course, well aware that there had been several other attempts at providing an "introductory" text. However our teaching experience indicated that, for one reason or another, they were not well suited for the clinician-to-be. Too often the introductory text turned out to be far too advanced for the introductory student, assuming more depth in mathematics, biology, and physics than our students possessed. In a sense, we set out to write an introductory text that laid the foundation for some other "introductory" texts. We especially felt that sophisticated mathematics should not be included in the text, and that those mathematical concepts that were necessary should be explained in plain English.

Since the great majority of our students ultimately become clinicians, we chose to include some basic clinical material in the text. This, we felt, would provide a sense of relevancy and a good transition from the purely physical and physiological to the clinical application.

Perhaps the most difficult task in writing a text of this type is to maintain the material at the introductory level and to keep the continuity of the book flowing from chapter to chapter. We often found it easier to write too much and in greater detail than was necessary for a first-level course. Therefore, the major goal of our editing was to limit ourselves to the basic concepts in hearing science.

We feel that the final product of our efforts represents a well-balanced approach to the study of hearing science for the introductory student. The book is comprehensive, but not so complex that it occupies the student's mind with unnecessary detail. The chapters were purposely limited to moderate length to enhance learning and motivation.

At the conclusion of each chapter there is a series of study questions with answers to assist the student in evaluating his or her learning of the material. There is also an annotated list of suggested readings from easily available sources at the conclusion of each chapter to assist readers who would like to know more about a particular topic. The glossaries at the ends of the chapters are meant to help the student in identifying the main concepts and terms. The glossary terms are often in somewhat greater detail than the discussion in the chapter; this should expand learning and provide a precise definition for reference. We feel that proper use of the post-chapter materials will add substantially to the effective use of this textbook.

We would like to take this opportunity to thank those people whose efforts contributed to the completion of this manuscript. Toby Deutsch painstakingly proofread the manuscript, and Judy Pilof typed it with great care. Ellen Pilof and Ellen Richards' assistance and comments were of great value.

We feel that the illustrations done by Valerie Aiksnoras are a high point in the book. Valerie, a speech pathologist from Stamford, Connecticut, labored beyond the call of duty, especially on some of the most intricate anatomical diagrams, which required imagination and creativity as well as technical skill.

Finally, we would like to publicly express our appreciation to J. Donald Harris, our mentor, who was instrumental in directing our careers.

L. J. D.
A. M. R.

*to*

*Our wives,*
   *Toby and Ellen*
*and our children,*
   *Allison and Barry*
      *and*
   *Brian and Michael*

# ELEMENTARY
# HEARING SCIENCE

# PART I
## SOUND
## AND
## ITS MEASUREMENT

# CHAPTER 1
# The Nature
# of Sound

Perhaps the first and most fundamental question that a professor may ask in an introductory hearing science class is, "What is sound?" At first, students usually have some general notion of what sound is—it is vibration. This, however, is often where the knowledge of sound stops. Sound is vibration, but vibration of what? In this chapter we will address ourselves to describing the nature of vibration and how sound is produced. The approach to the topic is nonmathematical and practical. We will also see how various aspects of sounds are measured.

## SOUND

### Overview

People find themselves constantly surrounded by a myriad of different types of sounds. Although these sounds may seem different to us and some may be more pleasing or meaningful than others, they all share certain common characteristics. If we were to investigate each sound individually we would see that there are four requisite conditions common to all sounds that are heard.

The first condition for the production of sound is that there must be an energy source. The source of energy may take on many different forms. It may be a finger plucking the string of a guitar, a hammer striking a nail into a piece of wood, or the force of air being expelled from the lungs past the vocal folds. As these examples imply, an energy source, in and of itself, will not produce a sound unless it is applied to some object. That object, in turn, must be capable of vibration. That is, if an object is to act as a vibrator it must be capable of moving in a to and fro manner around its original rest position.

We have seen so far that for sound to be produced there must be a source of energy, and this energy must be applied to a vibrator. How then is this vibration moved from the vibrator to our ears? The answer, of course, is that a medium must be interposed between the two. The medium

3

must be composed of molecules that are also capable of vibration. The most familiar medium through which sound travels is air. However, sound may also travel through water (or other liquids), through other gases in addition to air, and even through solids. The most important point to be made here is that the third element required for sound transmission is a medium. Sound will not travel if a medium is not interposed between the vibrator and the ear. In this regard, a favorite question to ask students is whether or not people can converse in a normal manner on the moon. The answer is no. Since there is no atmosphere on the moon, there is no medium between the speakers. Hence, sound cannot be transmitted in the usual way. Under these circumstances, if two persons tried to communicate with each other they would have to rely on radio transmissions.

Last, the final element necessary for sound is a receptor, the ear, which is capable of receiving, interpreting, and utilizing the sound.


## VIBRATION

### Simple Harmonic Motion

We have seen that vibration is the key factor in the production of sound. Vibration occurs when a body is disturbed by an external force so that it moves in a to and fro manner around its original point of rest. In order for the body to move in a back and forth manner, it must possess certain physical properties. For one, the body must be composed of material that has the property of *elasticity*. Elasticity is considered to be a restoring force, or the ability of the material to assume its original position once the force has been removed. In other words, the greater the elasticity (or restoring force), the greater the ability of the body to get back to its original shape. The second physical feature that a vibrating body must possess is *inertia*. Inertia is the tendency of a body to remain in motion once it is set in motion, or for the body to remain at rest if undisturbed. Simply stated, inertia is the ability of a body to continue doing what it has been doing.

Elasticity and inertia interact with each other during the process of vibration. Let's see how this occurs. Figure 1.1 shows a one-stringed guitar. Although we wouldn't expect this instrument to work well in producing music, it illustrates how vibration occurs. If we do not touch the string, it will remain at its rest point (position 1), or in its equilibrium state. If we move the string to position 2 and release it, the vibration process begins. When we first release the string its elasticity is high because it has been displaced from its rest position. This restoring force causes the string to move back. Once the rest position is reached, the inertia is high and this causes the string to move through its equilibrium point and in the opposite direction. As the string moves away from the rest

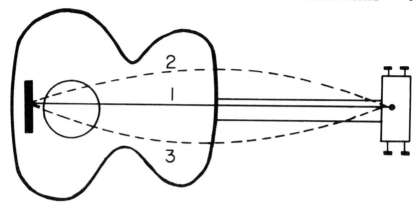

Figure 1.1.    Interaction of elasticity and inertia in vibration.

position, elasticity once again increases until its force exceeds the inertia at position 3; when this occurs the string will travel back toward the rest position again. The most important point to be made here is that inertia and elasticity act to oppose each other in the process of vibration. When inertia is high, elasticity is low, and vice versa. Vibrations of this sort will not be sustained for extended periods of time because the excursions of the string are reduced by frictional forces, and the vibration eventually stops. The process by which this reduction occurs is known as *damping*.

Although all vibration consists of back and forth motion, the manner in which this motion occurs over time may differ. Generally, vibration may take one of two forms, *periodic* or *aperiodic*. In periodic vibration, the motion of the vibrating body is predictable, and it occurs over and over again in the same manner. The motion of the guitar string in Figure 1.1 is periodic in that the string moves over and over again in the same way, and it takes the same time to complete each successive to and fro movement. Another name for this is *simple harmonic motion* (SHM). Sounds that are produced by simple harmonic motion have a tonal character and are referred to as *pure tones*. A tuning fork, for example, produces a pure tone since the tines vibrate in simple harmonic motion.

At this point, let's look at the most basic features of simple harmonic motion. Figure 1.2 shows a pendulum. The motion that a pendulum goes through over time is a classic example of simple harmonic motion. Once the pendulum is set in motion, the weight will swing back and forth in a repeatable manner, always taking the same time to complete one complete cycle or 1 *Hertz* (Hz).

To illustrate what a complete cycle consists of, let's set our pendulum in motion. If we arbitrarily begin our cycle when the pendulum is at its rest point (point A), the weight would have to first swing out to point B, back through point A to point C, and then back to point A once again in order

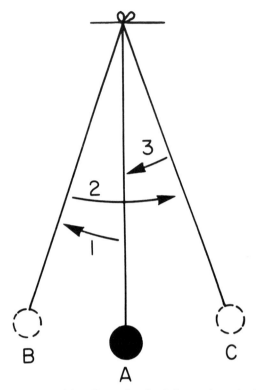

Figure 1.2.    A pendulum illustrating simple harmonic motion (SHM).

to complete one cycle. The time it takes to complete one cycle remains unchanged as long as the pendulum remains in motion.

How might we graph the motion of our pendulum over time? To do this, let's use our imaginations for a moment. Figure 1.3 shows the pendulum. The string has been attached to a horizontal bar that is capable of moving upward at a constant rate of speed. Imagine that the ball of the pendulum will somehow leave a trail as it swings through one cycle in its upward journey. As you can see in Figure 1.3, the resulting pattern is familiar to many of us; it is a *sine wave*.

**PURE TONES**

In Figure 1.4 we have redrawn the sine wave seen in Figure 1.3, but this time in the more familiar horizontal plane. Let's now look at some of the properties of sine waves. Remember that any vibrating body that moves in a simple and periodic way (i.e., SHM) can be plotted as a sine wave over time. Also remember that the sound produced by such a vibrating source has a definite tonal quality and, in fact, is referred to as a *pure tone*. Pure tone stimuli are extremely important in testing the hearing

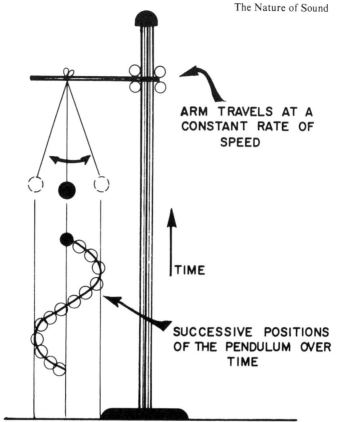

ARM TRAVELS AT A
CONSTANT RATE OF
SPEED

TIME

SUCCESSIVE POSITIONS
OF THE PENDULUM OVER
TIME

Figure 1.3.    Pendular motion over time.

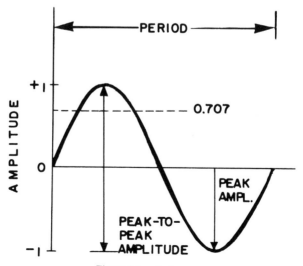

Figure 1.4.    A sine wave.

mechanism. Pure tones may be produced mechanically using tuning forks or they may be electronically generated. The fundamental diagnostic instrument for hearing tests, the audiometer, produces and controls several aspects of pure tones.

## Frequency

*Frequency* (*F*) represents one of the primary properties of pure tones. Frequency equals the number of completed cycles of vibration that occur in a 1-second time period. The unit of frequency is the Hertz (Hz). For example, if 20 completed vibrations occur in 1 second, the frequency is 20 Hz. If 1000 vibrations occur in 1 second the frequency is 1000 Hz. Frequency may also be expressed in kiloHertz (kHz) by dividing the number of Hertz by 1000. For example, a 1000-Hz tone may also be expressed as 1.0 kHz, a 2000-Hz tone as 2.0 kHz, and a 4500-Hz tone as 4.5 kHz.

The range of frequencies that humans are capable of hearing generally falls within the limits of 20 Hz and 20,000 Hz (20 kHz). As we will see in subsequent chapters, our sensitivity to all frequencies in the hearing range is not the same. We are most sensitive to frequencies falling between 1000 Hz and 3000 Hz, and less sensitive both above and below these frequencies.

The frequency of a pure tone is closely related to the perception of pitch. In general, the higher the frequency of the tone, the higher the perceived pitch. The exact relationship between frequency and perceived pitch is discussed at length in Chapter 12.

## Amplitude

In general, amplitude refers to the distance that a vibrator moves during vibration. The greater the distance from the rest position, the greater the amplitude. We see from Figure 1.4, however, that the amplitude of the sine wave is in a state of continuous variation. One moment the amplitude is at the zero crossing line (rest position) and the next moment it is somewhere between the rest position and the maximum displacement points. For this reason, there are several ways to specify the amplitude of a sine wave. *Peak amplitude* refers to the maximum momentary displacement obtained by the vibrating source. In the case of a sine wave, the peak amplitude occurs twice in a cycle. It occurs once when the vibrator reaches its maximum displacement in one direction (+1 in Figure 1.4), and again when the maximum displacement is reached in the opposite direction (−1 in Figure 1.4). *Peak-to-peak amplitude*, as the name implies, equals the distance between the maximum displacement points in both directions around the rest position. In the case of a sine wave, the peak-to-peak amplitude is simply twice the peak amplitude. *Instantaneous amplitude* is the amplitude that the wave assumes at any moment in time.

The most useful way of specifying the overall amplitude of a sine wave is in terms of its *effective level*. This value is a statistical average of all the amplitudes within the waveform at each instant in time. We should note, however, that the effective level of a sine wave is not simply a straight average of all the instantaneous amplitudes. If we do this, the obtained level would, of course, then be zero. This would occur because a sine wave extends as much above the baseline (0) as it does below the baseline. For this reason, the effective level is taken as the *root-mean-square* (*RMS*) value. What is done here is that all the momentary amplitudes in the wave are first squared (this eliminates all the negative numbers); an average value is then obtained. The square root of the average is the RMS value. In the case of a sine wave, the RMS value, or effective level, is equal to the peak amplitude multiplied by 0.707.

Most measurement instruments found in the hearing science laboratory or audiology clinic measure the RMS values of pure tones. For example, voltmeters are most often calibrated in volts RMS. Similarly, *sound level meters* respond to the RMS values of the measured sound levels.

The amplitude of a pure tone is closely related to the perception of loudness. In general, the greater the amplitude, the louder the tone sounds. The exact relationship between the amplitude of a tone and loudness perception is discussed in detail in Chapter 12.

### Period

The period of an object that moves in simple harmonic motion is the time it takes to complete one cycle of vibration. The period then is the reciprocal of frequency or, mathematically speaking, 1/frequency. For example, the period of a 1000-Hz tone is 1/1000, or one one-thousandth of a second. In other words, if 1000 Hz occur in 1 second, then it takes the tone 1/1000 second to complete 1 Hz.

### Phase

The phase of an object that vibrates in SHM represents that portion of a cycle that has elapsed at any instant in time, relative to some arbitrary starting point. Phase is expressed in degrees, and the number of degrees contained within one completed cycle is 360. Thus, the *phase angle* at any point during a cycle may vary between 0° and 360°. The concept of phase is derived from the close relationship between simple harmonic motion and *projected circular motion*. Let's take a closer look at this relationship.

Figure 1.5 shows a wheel that can be turned at a constant rate of speed. A small hole is drilled at the edge of the wheel into which a thin metal rod is inserted; the rod is free to pivot as the wheel rotates. The distance between the center of the wheel and the hole, R, is equal to the radius of a circle. The other end of the rod is attached to a pen assembly

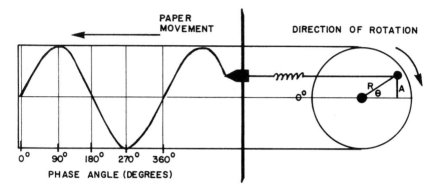

Figure 1.5.   Phase of a sine wave.

that can move vertically up and down a shaft. In order to make this machine work properly we have to put a spring between the rod and the pen assembly to maintain constant tension as the wheel rotates. As the wheel rotates the pen assembly moves. In fact, the position of the pen at any instant in time is exactly equal to the height of the hole above or below the center of the circle (distance A in Figure 1.5). If the wheel rotates one complete cycle (360°), the pen assembly will move through one complete cycle of vibration. For example, if we begin one rotation of the wheel when the hole is at the 0° point, the pen will move first in one direction, back through the baseline and in the opposite direction, and then back to the baseline again. In other words, 360° of rotation can be projected as one cycle of simple harmonic motion. If we were now to move a piece of paper past the pen at a constant rate of speed, the obtained pattern would be a sine wave. Each point on the sine wave could then be specified as the number of degrees that elapsed in the cycle. Specifically, each point on the sine wave would equal the angle at which the radius met the baseline, $\theta$, which is referred to as the *phase angle*. The maximum amplitude of the sine wave would, of course, equal the length of the radius.

**Phase Difference**

As the term implies, a *phase difference* refers to the difference in phase angles between two different vibrating sources. For the sake of simplicity, let us make both sources pure tones of the same frequency and amplitude. We can represent the motion of both vibrating sources that produce the tones in much the same manner as in Figure 1.5. This time, however, there are two small holes at the edge of the wheel, one for each of the tones (Figure 1.6). Two pens are attached to the holes by separate rods. The distance in degrees between the holes along the perimeter of the wheel represents the phase difference between the tones. In this case, the figure shows a phase difference of 90°. In other words, one tone lags the other (B lags A) by one-quarter of a cycle. As the wheel rotates at a constant rate both pens will now move in simple harmonic motion. Pen B, however, will always lag behind pen A by 90°. The resulting pattern on the paper that moves past the pens is seen in Figure 1.6. It shows that whenever one vibrator is at the zero crossing line (equilibrium point) the other vibrator is at the point of maximum displacement. For example at point 1, A is at the equilibrium point while B is at the point of maximum displacement in the positive (upward) direction. At point 2, B is at the zero crossing point while A is at the maximum displacement point in the negative direction.

The term *in phase* refers to a condition where a 0° phase difference exists between two vibrating sources. In other words, both vibrators assume identical phase angles at every instant in time. The term *phase opposition* refers to a condition in which the vibrating sources are 180° out of phase. Under these circumstances the vibrators always assume opposite positions relative to the baseline level. Figure 1.7 illustrates both the in phase and phase opposition conditions. Since the amplitudes of the vibrators are assumed to be equal, the pattern that we see for the phase opposition condition is one of equal, but reversed, displacements at each instant in time. In other words, if two tones are sounded, and they are in phase opposition, and they are of equal intensity and frequency, the result will be complete cancellation.

### COMPLEX VIBRATION: COMPLEX TONES AND NOISE

Until now our discussion of vibration has been principally concerned with simple harmonic motion (SHM) and the tonal nature of the sounds it

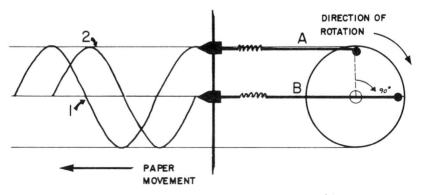

Figure 1.6.   Phase difference of 90° (one-quarter cycle).

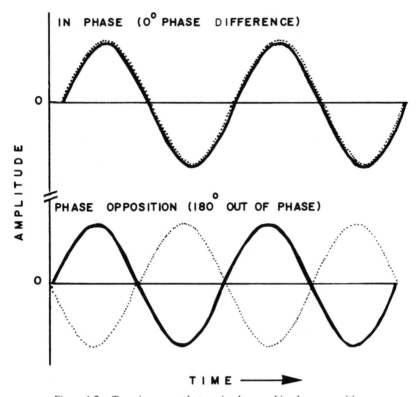

Figure 1.7.   Two sine waves that are in phase and in phase opposition.

produces. The scientific usefulness of pure tones is indisputable. Pure tones are used extensively for both measurement and calibration purposes in the acoustics/psychoacoustics laboratory, and they are used to determine the degree of hearing impairment in the audiology clinic. Pure tones, however, are not often encountered in everyday situations. Most sounds that we hear in ordinary life are of a complex nature; their vibrating sources do not move in a simple back and forth motion. Two types of complex vibration are of interest to us. The first, called *complex periodic vibration*, like SHM, is periodic in that it produces a waveform that repeats itself over and over again in time. However, the pattern produced by complex periodic vibration is something other than a sine wave. *Aperiodic vibration*, as the name implies, does not produce repeatable patterns of vibration. The sounds produced by complex periodic vibration are known as *complex tones*, whereas the sounds produced by aperiodic vibration are simply referred to as *noise*.

Before considering the composition of complex tones and noise, it is important to understand the concept of *spectrum*. The spectrum of any sound is a plot which shows the amplitude of each frequency component in the sound. Spectrum should not be confused with *waveform*. The waveform of a sound is a plot that shows the amplitude of the sound at each instant in *time*. Consider for a moment the spectrum and waveform of a simple sound—a pure tone. Figure 1.8(A) shows the waveform of a 1000-Hz tone. Figure 1.8(B) shows the spectrum for the same sound. The waveform seen in A is already familiar. The vibrating source that produces the sound yields a sine wave over time with a period of 1/1000 second. The spectrum of the tone is simply a straight line, or *line spectrum*, at 1000 Hz. In other words, the entire energy of the sound is concentrated at one frequency only, 1000 Hz. The height of the line corresponds to the amplitude of the tone so that the higher the line, the greater the amplitude.

Complex tones are produced when two or more pure tones are sounded together. The resulting waveform is not a sine wave, but it is a pattern that repeats itself over and over again in time. Figure 1.9 shows the waveform of two pure tones, where one is twice the frequency of the other. Also shown in the figure is the combined waveform (C) which results when both tones are sounded together. The combined waveform is different from both of the component tones, but it is periodic in that it repeats itself regularly.

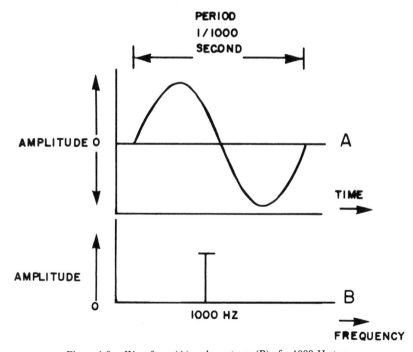

Figure 1.8.   Waveform (A) and spectrum (B) of a 1000-Hz tone.

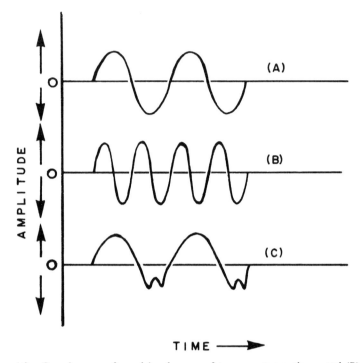

Figure 1.9.   Complex wave formed by the sum of two pure tones, the second (B) being twice the frequency of the first (A).

The waveform of a complex tone depends upon the phases and amplitudes of the individual component frequencies. The amplitude of a complex wave at any instant in time is equal to the algebraic sum of the component waves. As the phase relationships and amplitudes change, so does the appearance of the combined waveform. The resultant pattern that we saw for the two pure tones in Figure 1.9 then represents only one of many patterns that might have been obtained for the same two pure tone frequencies.

Figure 1.10 shows the spectrum of the complex tone seen in Figure 1.9. Remember that one tone was twice the frequency of the other. Suppose that the lower frequency tone was 1000 Hz and the higher frequency tone was 2000 Hz. The spectrum is simply two lines, one at each of the component frequencies. In other words, all the energy in the sound was concentrated at only two points along the auditory spectrum. Notice that in this case the amplitude of the 2000-Hz tone is less than that of the 1000-Hz tone. All complex tones, regardless of the number of component frequencies, have *line spectra*. Stated in another way, all complex tones may be broken down into a series of discrete pure tone components of varying amplitudes and phases.

We have seen to this point that a complex tone consists of two or more frequencies that are sounded together. Musical tones are, in fact, complex tones whose frequencies are related to each other in a *harmonic series*. If we represent the lowest frequency, or *fundamental*, in a harmonic series as $f$, then the component frequencies are $2f$, $3f$, $4f$, and so on. The component frequencies are integral multiples of the fundamental, and are known as *harmonics*. For example, if the fundamental were 100 Hz, the second harmonic would be 200 Hz; the third harmonic, 300 Hz; the fourth harmonic, 400 Hz; and so on up the frequency scale. Although many instruments may play the same note on the musical scale (this corresponds to the fundamental frequency), each instrument possesses its own special sound qualities. This quality, or *timbre*, is derived from varying amplitude patterns of the harmonic frequencies. In other words, the amplitudes of the harmonics vary in relative intensity from one instrument to another.

We noted earlier that aperiodic vibration is usually referred to as noise. We usually associate noise with something that should be reduced or eliminated, and this is true in many cases. In other cases, however, noise signals provide us with important information. For example, many of the consonant sounds of speech that we produce and hear are, in fact, noise. They are produced by the individual constricting his vocal tract in one way or another, which then creates a turbulent flow of air.

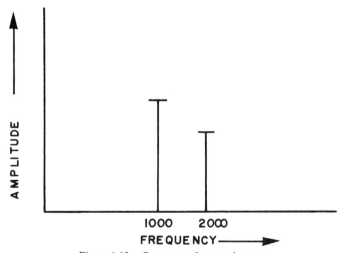

Figure 1.10.   Spectrum of a complex tone.

The main feature of aperiodic vibration is that the sounds it produces do not have tonal qualities. If we were to plot the waveform of such a sound, it would be irregular with no repeatable patterns.

In the audiology clinic we use various types of noise to eliminate the possibility of *cross-hearing*. Cross-hearing occurs sometimes in hearing tests when the test signal is actually heard in the ear we are not testing. In order to conduct a reliable and accurate hearing examination, the ears must be measured in isolation from each other. When cross-hearing is suspected, the audiologist can introduce either *white noise* or *narrowband noise* into the non-test ear while measuring hearing function on the test side. We shall look further into cross-hearing in Chapter 11 (Masking).

White noise sounds like steam escaping from a radiator. It is composed of all the pure tone frequencies in the audible spectrum sounded together with no regard to phase. Figure 1.11 shows both the waveform (A) and the spectrum (B) of white noise. Notice that the waveform shows no repeatable pattern over time. The spectrum of white noise is flat. In other words, all the frequency components in the noise, although produced without regard to phase, are of equal amplitudes. Thus, white noise has a continuous and *flat spectrum*.

Narrowband noise is similar to white noise in that its component frequencies sound without regard to phase. As the name implies, however, the frequencies that comprise narrowband noise are restricted in their range. Figure 1.12 shows the waveform (A) and spectrum (B) of a narrow band of noise. Notice that the waveform is similar to that of white noise. However, the spectrum differs from that of white noise in that all the acoustic energy falls only within specified *noise band limits*.

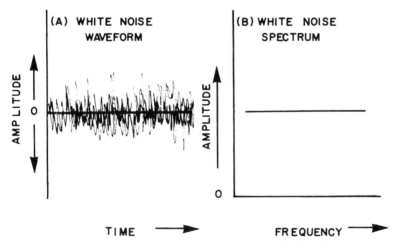

Figure 1.11.   Waveform (A) and spectrum (B) of white noise.

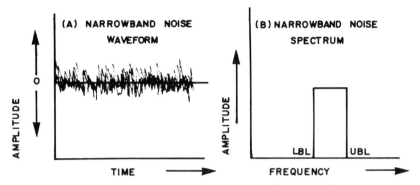

Figure 1.12.    Waveform (A) and spectrum (B) of narrowband noise.

The *lower band limit* (specified in Hz) is found at the lower frequency limit of the noise band, and the *upper band limit* (also in Hz) falls at the higher frequency limit of the noise band. The *bandwidth* of the noise is the difference (in Hz) between the upper and lower band limits. For example, if the lower band limit were 1000 Hz and the upper band limit were 3000 Hz, the bandwidth would be 2000 Hz. As was the case for white noise, narrowband noise has a flat and continuous spectrum. Thus, all the component frequencies are of equal amplitudes.

### SOUND WAVES

Sound cannot be produced unless a medium is interposed between the source of vibration and the ear. The most familiar medium to us is air. When vibration falls within the range of human hearing (20 to 20,000 Hz) and this vibration is conveyed to our ears, a *sound wave* has been produced.

To understand what a sound wave is we must first begin with a vibrator. For the sake of simplicity, let's use a tuning fork as an example, to produce vibration that is simple and periodic. If the tuning fork is struck, the tines move back and forth. When this occurs air particles (molecules) that surround the tines move back and forth. Since air is an elastic medium (the air molecules possess the properties of elasticity and inertia), each molecule mimics the original pattern of vibration. The effect of the vibrator is not limited only to those air particles in the immediate vicinity of the tines of the tuning fork, because each particle acts as a separate vibrator which then causes adjacent particles to vibrate. The end result is a wave of air particle movement which emanates in all directions from the original source of vibration. The speed of a sound wave in air is generally about 1100 feet per second (335 meters per second).

Let's now look in a bit more detail at the sound wave produced by the tuning fork. Figure 1.13 shows the tuning fork in a state of vibration. The right-hand tine has been labeled with the letters R and C. R represents the condition when the tine is in a state of inward motion, and C represents the condition when the tine is in a state of outward motion.

When the tine is in a state of outward motion, it compresses many air particles in front of it. This *compression* state represents a small, but measurable, increase in air pressure. When the tine moves back through the equilibrium point to the R position, it compresses the air particles in the opposite direction. In the meantime, however, the air particles in the original area of compression have been allowed to spread apart. This is a state of *rarefaction.* It represents a slight decrease in air pressure. As the tuning fork continues to vibrate, the same group of molecules will alternately go through compressions and rarefactions. An area that in one instant is in a state of compression will, in the next instant, be in a state of rarefaction. These alternating conditions of compression and rarefaction will travel away from the tuning fork through the surrounding air. In sum, the sound wave produced by a tuning fork is actually a wave of alternate increases (compressions) and decreases (rarefactions) in air pressure which emanate from the original vibrating source.

One important point needs to be emphasized: an individual air particle that is either in a state of compression or rarefaction does not travel all the way from the sound source to the ear. The individual particles move only short distances and collide with adjacent air particles. This process, by which the vibratory energy is transferred from one particle to another, forms the sound wave.

An important question we might ask ourselves is, "What is the distance between successive compressions (or rarefactions) in space?" This distance is known as the *wavelength.* Wavelength (denoted by the Greek letter lambda ($\lambda$)) is equal to the speed of sound divided by frequency, or:

$$\text{Wavelength } (\lambda) = \text{Speed of sound/Frequency}$$

For example, if the tuning fork vibrated at 1000 Hz, the wavelength would equal:

$$\text{Wavelength } (\lambda) = \frac{1100 \text{ feet/second}}{1000 \text{ Hz}} = 1.1 \text{ feet, or, metrically,}$$

$$\text{Wavelength } (\lambda) = \frac{335 \text{ meters/second}}{1000 \text{ Hz}} = 0.34 \text{ meters/second}$$

In other words, the distance in space between successive compressions (or rarefactions) would be 1.1 feet, or its metric equivalent of 0.34 meters, for the 1000-Hz tone. Therefore, as the frequency becomes higher the wavelength becomes shorter.

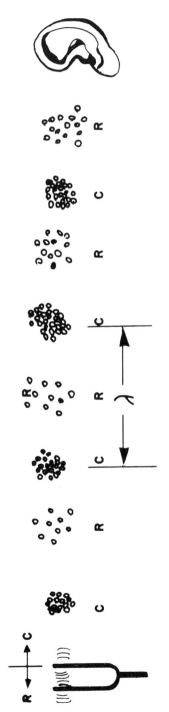

Figure 1.13. Sound wave produced by a vibrating tuning fork.

Note that the intensity of sound is reduced as it travels away from the sound source. This occurs because of frictional forces between adjacent molecules, which cause some of the sound energy to be converted to heat. The law that governs this reduction in intensity is called the *inverse square law*.

## SOUND INTENSITY AND THE DECIBEL

The final important area in the physics of sound that we must cover is sound *intensity*, and its unit of measurement, the *decibel*. The understanding and use of the decibel is essential in audiology and hearing science. The concepts involved are straightforward and relatively simple, even if you have a limited background in physics and mathematics.

Chapter 2 is devoted entirely to the concept of intensity and the use of decibels. It is written so that you will need no more mathematical sophistication than long division.

## GLOSSARY

*amplitude*—The amplitude of a sound wave is related to the distance that the sound-producing body (the vibrator) moves during vibration. The greater the distance from the point of rest, the greater the amplitude. *Instantaneous amplitude* refers to the excursion distance at any point in time, whereas *peak amplitude* refers to the greatest point of displacement. The *RMS (root-mean-square) amplitude* is a statistical average of all amplitudes at all times. (See *root-mean-square amplitude*.)

*aperiodic vibration*—Vibration that is not repeatable over time. Sounds produced by aperiodic vibration are generally classified as noise.

*audiometer*—An instrument for measuring hearing thresholds. Hearing measurements are typically obtained for both pure tone and speech signals. The stimuli produced by audiometers are presented to the listener through a pair of earphones, a bone conduction vibrator, or loudspeaker. The level of the stimulus is controlled by the examiner until a threshold level is obtained. The results are plotted on an audiogram.

*bandwidth*—The frequency difference between the lower and upper noise band limits. More generally, however, the bandwidth of any device or system is the range of frequencies within which the performance of the device or system remains above a specified level.

*complex tone*—A periodic sound wave that consists of a fundamental frequency combined with other sine wave components at different frequencies.

*compression*—Occurs when the air particles are pushed together. This condition increases the resting air pressure.

*effective level*—See *root-mean-square amplitude.*

*elasticity*—The property of a medium or a body that enables it to return to its original shape after it has been deformed. Elasticity may be considered a restoring force; the greater the elasticity, the more resistant the medium or body to deformation.

*frequency*—The number of complete cycles that a periodically vibrating source passes through in a 1-second time period. Frequency is expressed in Hertz (Hz).

*fundamental frequency*—The lowest frequency component in a complex tone. (See *complex tone* and *harmonic series.*)

*harmonics*—Pure tone components of a complex tone that are integral multiples of the fundamental frequency. (See *fundamental frequency, complex tone,* and *harmonic series.*)

*harmonic series*—A complex sound wave that consists of a fundamental frequency together with other pure tone components at integral multiples of the fundamental. (See *complex tone.*)

*Hertz*—The unit of measurement for frequency. The term *Hertz* was named in honor of Heinrich Hertz (1857–1894), an important German physicist. Hz is synonymous with the formerly used expression cycles per second (cps). (See *frequency.*)

*inertia*—The ability of a body to continue doing what it has been doing. If the body is at rest, it will tend to remain at rest. If the body is in motion, it will tend to remain in motion.

*in phase*—The condition in which two waveforms of the same frequency coincide exactly in their phase angles (phase difference). That is, both waves correspond exactly in their minimums and maximums at the same instants in time. (See *phase angle* and *phase difference.*)

*instantaneous amplitude*—The amplitude of a vibrating source at any instant in time. (See *amplitude.*)

*intensity*—The amount of acoustic energy that passes through a unit of area in a given time span. Intensity may be measured in units of power or pressure directly, but more frequently intensity is measured in decibels, which are logarithmic ratios.

*narrowband*—Noise that is restricted in its frequency range. The spectrum of narrowband noise is continuous (no gaps), and the frequency components are all of equal amplitudes. Like white noise, there is no regard to phase of the pure tone components. (See *white noise.*)

*noise*—Any undesired sound.

*noise band limits*—Those frequencies below or above which there is no appreciable noise energy. In practice, the band limit frequency is often taken as that point where the energy content is 3 dB below the average energy in the pass band.

*peak amplitude*—The maximum instantaneous displacement of a vibrating source from its point of rest. (See *amplitude.*)

*peak-to-peak amplitude*—The amplitude of a vibrating source, measured from the maximum positive peak to the maximum negative peak.

*period*—The time it takes to complete one cycle of vibration. Period is defined as $1/f$, where $f$ is the frequency of vibration. The period of a 1000-Hz tone is then $1/1000$, or one one-thousandth of a second.

*periodic vibration*—Vibration that repeats itself regularly over time. Both pure tones and complex tones are sounds produced by periodic vibration. (See *pure tone* and *complex tone.*)

*phase angle*—That portion of a cycle (Hz) which has elapsed at a given instant in time, relative to some arbitrary starting point. Because of the relation between simple harmonic motion (SHM) and projected circular motion, the phase angle may vary between 0° and 360°. (See *simple harmonic motion.*)

*phase difference*—The difference in phase angles between two periodic waveforms at any instant in time, relative to some arbitrary starting point. For example, if two 1000-Hz tones are started one-fourth cycle apart, their phase difference will be 90°. (See *phase angle.*)

*phase opposition*—The condition in which two waveforms of the same frequency are exactly one-half of a cycle (180°) out of phase. That is, when one wave is at its maximum value, the other is, at the same instant, at its minimum value. Thus, the two waveforms always assume opposite but equal positions relative to the baseline. (See *phase difference.*)

*pure tone*—A sound with a definite tonal quality. The waveform of the vibrating body that produces the pure tone is a sine wave. The frequency (in Hz) of a pure tone represents the completed number of cycles the vibrating source passes through in a 1-sec time period.

*rarefaction*—Occurs when air particles are separated. This condition results in a decrease in the resting air pressure.

*root-mean-square (RMS) amplitude*—Represents the *effective amplitude* of the source. Mathematically, the RMS amplitude is equal to the square root of the mean of all the squared instantaneous amplitudes. For the case of a sine wave, the RMS amplitude equals 0.707 times the peak amplitude. (See *amplitude.*)

*simple harmonic motion*—A symmetrical to and fro motion of a body over a rest position. When the amplitudes of the body are plotted as a function of time, the resulting pattern is a sine wave. Pure tones are produced by simple harmonic motion.

*sound level meter*—An instrument that measures sound levels in decibels with a specific reference of 0.0002 dyne/cm². A sound level meter typically consists of a microphone, amplifier, output meter or digital display, and several frequency-weighting networks. The purpose of the networks is to simulate the response characteristics of the normal human ear.

*spectrum*—A plot showing the frequencies and amplitudes of the individual components of the wave. A *line spectrum* is one in which the energy in the wave is at only one or more discrete frequencies (a pure tone or a complex tone). A *continuous spectrum* is one in which there is a continuous and unbroken band of frequencies. Spectrum is also used to denote a range of frequencies that possess a common characteristic, such as the audio-frequency spectrum.

*timbre*—The character of a musical tone that distinguishes one musical instrument from another. Timbre depends upon the relative intensities of the harmonic frequencies produced by each instrument.

*waveform*—A plot that shows the instantaneous amplitudes of the signal over time.

*wavelength*—The wavelength of a periodic sound wave (i.e., a pure tone) is the distance in space between two corresponding points (phases) in two consecutive cycles. Wavelength is related to the velocity of sound and frequency by the formula: $\lambda$ (wavelength) = $V$ (velocity)/$F$ (frequency).

*white noise*—consists of a continuous spectrum across the auditory range. Although the amplitudes of all the frequency components that comprise the noise are equal, there is no regard to the phases of the frequency components.

## SUGGESTED READINGS FOR FURTHER STUDY

Davis, H., and S. R. Silverman. 1978. *Hearing and Deafness*, Chapter 2. 4th Ed. Holt, Rinhart & Winston, New York.
A good introductory overview.
Tonndorf, J. 1965. Acoustics. In A. Glorig (ed.), *Audiometry*. Williams & Wilkins Company, Baltimore.
A thorough introduction.
Van Bergeijk, W. A., J. R. Pierce, and E. E. David. 1960. *Waves and the Ear*. Doubleday & Company, Inc., New York.
An easy-to-read introduction.

## STUDY QUESTIONS

1. The primary unit of frequency is the _____.
2. The number of completed cycles in a 1-second time period is known as _____.
3. The distance a vibrating body moves from its point of rest is known as _____.
4. The _____ of a wave is equal to the time needed to complete one cycle.
5. The type of vibration that will produce a pure tone is known as _____.
6. Two tones that are in phase opposition (180°) will result in _____.
7. As frequency increases, the wavelength of a pure tone will _____.
8. The waveform of a pure tone is plotted as a _____.
9. The lowest frequency in a harmonic series is known as the _____.
10. A sound composed of several pure tones is known as a _____.

# CHAPTER 2
# Sound Intensity and the Decibel

*Intensity* is the physical measure of what we perceive as the loudness of a sound. The greater the intensity of sound, the louder it normally appears to be.

Chapter 1 explained that a sound wave is created by rapid vibrations of air particles that travel outward from the source of vibration (for example, a tuning fork). When these particles are in a state of compression, there is an increase in air pressure; when they are in a state of rarefaction, there is a decrease in pressure.

In audiology, we normally measure the intensity of a sound in terms of sound (acoustic) pressure. The greater the pressure change, the greater the intensity of a sound. The ear is very sensitive to changes in sound pressure, and a small change in pressure (intensity) will result in an increase (or decrease) in loudness sensation. The relationship between intensity and loudness is not a simple one, and it is discussed in greater depth in Chapter 12.

The intensity of a pure tone is measured by the amplitude of the sine wave. Greater amplitude represents greater particle displacement and, therefore, greater sound intensity.

Figure 2.1 shows two pure tones of equal frequency and phase, but pure tone *a* has a smaller amplitude than pure tone *b*. If the two pure tones were played through a loudspeaker, they would have the same pitch, but *b* would seem louder than *a*.

Intensity is normally measured in sound pressure. For other scientific purposes, intensities can also be measured in terms of power, but that is rarely done in audiology. Physics tells us that pressure is created when a force is distributed over an area. In other words:

$$\text{Pressure} = \frac{\text{Force}}{\text{Area}}$$

A common unit of force used in sound measurement is the *dyne*. A square centimeter (cm²) is, of course, a unit of area. The unit of pressure we normally use is the dyne per centimeter square:

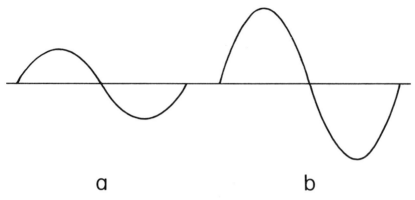

a                                b

Figure 2.1.   Two pure tones of the same frequency and phase, but of different intensities (amplitudes).

$$\frac{dyne}{cm^2}$$

Therefore, when we measure pressure in dynes/cm², we are, in fact, measuring the force of a sound vibration over a given unit of area.

## LINEAR AND LOGARITHMIC SCALES

The human ear is capable of hearing a very wide range of sound intensities. If we compare the softest sound that we can hear (about 0.0002 dyne/cm²) to the loudest sound we hear without pain (about 2000 dynes/cm²), the loud sound would be 10 million times the intensity of the soft sound.

Although it is possible to measure sound pressure in dynes/cm², it would force us to use very large numbers to describe a person's hearing levels—a patient might well have a hearing loss of 5 million dynes/cm². For this reason, it is never done in clinical practice. Normally, we measure intensity in a unit called the *decibel* (dB), which was named in honor of Alexander Graham Bell.

It is important to note that the decibel is a *logarithmic scale*, as opposed to a *linear scale*, which we usually deal with. In linear measurement, all units on the scale are the same size. Therefore, 1 inch to 2 inches on a ruler is exactly the same distance as 11 inches to 12 inches. An inch is an inch no matter where it lies on the ruler. Similarly, the difference between 2 pounds and 3 pounds is identical to the difference between 102 pounds and 103 pounds. Both inches and pounds are linear scales.

In a logarithmic scale, each unit in the scale is larger than the preceding unit. A good analogy is the geometric progression:

1,2,4,8,16,32,64 . . .

Table 2.1.  A comparison of pressure and decibel scales as intensity increases

| Linear scale: Pressure | Log scale: Decibels |
|---|---|
| 1 | 0 dB |
| 1 × 10 | 20 dB |
| 1 × 100 | 40 dB |
| 1 × 1000 | 60 dB |
| 1 × 10,000 | 80 dB |
| 1 × 100,000 | 100 dB |
| 1 × 1,000,000 | 120 dB |
| 1 × 10,000,000 | 140 dB |

In this series of numbers, the distance between units is not equal as we go up the scale, but gets progressively larger.

A common example of a logarithmic scale is the FM radio dial. As we go from left to right, the range of numbers that fits into the same distance (say 1 inch) is far greater. By using the logarithmic (log) scale on the FM dial, all the stations can fit into a much smaller space.

The use of a log scale, the decibel (dB), for hearing avoids very large numbers and allows us to describe the entire range of human hearing (10 million-fold in linear terms) as 0 dB to 140 dB.

Table 2.1 shows the relationship between increases in pressure, a linear scale, and the decibel, a logarithmic scale. In this table, we arbitrarily call the starting pressure "1" and make this equal to 0 dB.

Table 2.1 shows that a tenfold increase in pressure (linear) will always yield a 20-dB increase, no matter what the actual numbers happen to be. For example, a pressure change of 1 to 10 yields a 20-dB difference, as does the pressure ratio 10,000 to 100,000. We can conclude that, unlike a linear scale, the sizes of succeeding decibel units do not always equal each other. Therefore, a change from 1 to 2 dB is smaller than from 2 to 3 dB. The higher we go in the scale, the greater the amount of linear pressure change that is indicated by a 1-dB increase in intensity.

Although we are afforded the great convenience of describing human hearing from 0 dB to 140 dB, rather than being burdened with the arithmetic problems of much larger numbers, we are limited in other ways. Because the units are not linear, we cannot add or subtract decibels in the conventional manner, e.g., 10 dB + 10 dB does *not* equal 20 dB. Actually, whenever you double the pressure, you add only 6 dB:

$$10\,dB + 10\,dB = 16\,dB$$

and

$$50\,dB + 50\,dB = 56\,dB$$

Before continuing this discussion of logarithms and decibels, a few more basic concepts must be discussed in order to fully understand the nature of the decibel.

## ABSOLUTE AND RELATIVE SCALES

Although a more complete discussion of scaling is contained in the chapter on loudness and pitch (Chapter 12), the difference between absolute scales and relative scales is essential to the understanding of the decibel.

An *absolute scale* is one in which the zero point of the scale represents the absence of what is being measured. For example, 0 inches represents the absence of distance; something cannot be $-2$ inches long. Likewise, 0 pounds represents the absence of weight. Something can weigh 2 pounds less than something else, but it cannot weigh $-2$ pounds. In a *relative scale*, there is no true zero point; the zero value on the scale is arbitrarily chosen and must be agreed to by all users of the scale. An example of this is the temperature scale. In Celsius, $0°$ is arbitrarily chosen to equal the freezing point of water, and is the base of the scale. Unlike our absolute scales, however, it can be $-10°$ Celsius. In a relative scale, the zero point does not mean the absence of the measure; it is simply the base of the scale. Minus $10°$ Celsius means that the temperature measured is $10°$ colder than the freezing point of water, the arbitrary base of the Celsius scale. All relative scales must have an agreed-upon zero point, as does the Celsius scale; when using a relative scale, one is actually comparing the measured value to the base of the scale. Measured values that are less than the arbitrary zero will have negative numbers (like $-10°$), while values that are greater than the zero point will have positive numbers.

The decibel is a relative scale and therefore must have an arbitrary reference or zero point. Since we normally measure intensity in terms of sound pressure, and the approximate lower limit of human hearing is 0.0002 dyne/cm², this value is traditionally chosen for 0 dB. Whenever we use this base or reference point, we identify the measure with the suffix sound pressure level (SPL) in order to tell the user that the zero point of our decibel scale is 0.0002 dyne/cm². Therefore, if the intensity of a 1000-Hz tone is 50 dB SPL, we mean that it is 50 dB more intense than a 1000-Hz tone of 0 dB SPL (0.0002 dyne/cm²). In essence, we are saying that logarithmic scales with arbitrary zero points (relative scales) are ratios between the measured value and the base or reference point of the scale. This ratio of the measured value to the reference of the scale holds true for values smaller than 0.0002 dyne/cm² as well. If a pure tone has an intensity of $-10$ dB SPL, then it is 10 dB lower in intensity than the reference zero point.

We already know that the decibel scale is logarithmic. We also know that since it is a relative scale, it is based on a ratio. Another way of saying this is that the decibel is the log of the ratio between a measured intensity and a reference intensity which represents the zero point of the scale. To further explore this statement and the use of the dB, a basic working knowledge of logarithms is necessary. We will now take a few pages to review, in simple arithmetic terms, the concepts we will need.

## EXPONENTS AND LOGARITHMS

Only an elementary working knowledge of logarithms is needed to understand decibels, but it is important to understand each section before going on to the next.

In the arithmetic expression:

$$10^2$$

10 is referred to as the *base* and $^2$ as the exponent. A logarithm is the same as an exponent. *There is no difference.* Therefore, the log of $10^2$ (ten squared) is 2. Ten squared means:

$$10^2 = 10 \times 10 = 100$$

Since $10^2$ equals 100 and the log of $10^2$ is 2, the log of 100 must be 2.

$$10^3 = 10 \times 10 \times 10 = 1000$$

Since 1000, written in exponential form, is $10^3$, and the log is the same as the exponent, then the log of 1000 must be 3.

The log of 100,000 is 5:

$$10^5 = 10 \times 10 \times 10 \times 10 \times 10 = 100,000$$

A shortcut is that the log (or exponent) equals the number of zeros following the 1:

the log of 10 is 1
the log of 100 is 2
the log of 1000 is 3
the log of 10,000 is 4 . . .

In this chapter we always assume that the base used is 10. Other bases are sometimes used in mathematics, but rarely in relation to decibel measurements.

It is important to note that the log of 1 is *zero*:

$$10^0 = 1, \text{ therefore the log of } 1 = 0$$

This is easily confirmed since there are no zeros following the 1, and the log can be determined by counting the number of zeros that follow the 1.

## THE DECIBEL FORMULA

The formula, in terms of pressure, for the decibel is:

$$dB = 20 \times \log \frac{\text{pressure measured}}{\text{pressure reference}}$$

Remember that the decibel is a relative scale, and therefore requires a reference point. We said earlier that the normal pressure reference in auditory measurements is 0.0002 dyne/cm². We can now substitute this value in the formula:

$$dB = 20 \times \log \frac{\text{pressure measured}}{0.0002 \text{ dyne/cm}^2}$$

In order to solve this formula, we must insert the top number of the ratio (the pressure measured) and solve the ratio by dividing, then determine the logarithm of the resulting number, and multiply by 20. Let's take these steps one at a time with an example. Let's say that the pressure we measure is 2 dynes/cm², and we want to find out the number of decibels that this would equal in terms of pressure. First the ratio:

$$\frac{2 \text{ dynes/cm}^2}{0.0002 \text{ dyne/cm}^2}$$

Using long division, this is equal to 10,000:

$$0.0002 \overline{\smash{\big)}\,2.0000} = 2 \overline{\smash{\big)}\,\overset{\textstyle 10,000}{20,000}}$$

We know that the next step is to determine the log of 10,000 since the formula now reads:

$$dB = 20 \times \log 10,000$$

Looking back to our exercise in exponents, we know that 10,000 is the same as $10^4$:

$$10,000 = 10 \times 10 \times 10 \times 10 = 10^4$$

Since the log is the exponent, the log of 10,000 must be 4. Now our formula reads:

$$dB = 20 \times 4 \text{ or } \boxed{80 \text{ dB}}$$

Remember that we always use the suffix SPL when the reference point of our scale is 0.0002 dyne/cm², so the correct answer is:

$$80 \text{ dB SPL}$$

We can test our understanding by determining the number of dB SPL that would be generated by a sound pressure of 0.02 dyne/cm²:

$$\text{dB SPL} = 20 \times \log \frac{0.02 \text{ dyne/cm}^2}{0.0002 \text{ dyne/cm}^2}$$

*Step one: Solve the ratio by dividing.*

$$\frac{0.02}{0.0002} = 100$$

*Step two: Determine the logarithm by changing to exponential form.*

$$100 = 10^2$$

Therefore, the log of 100 is 2.

*Step three: Multiply by 20.*

$$\text{dB SPL} = 20 \times \log 100$$
$$\text{dB SPL} = 20 \times 2$$
$$\text{dB SPL} = 40$$

The answer is therefore    40 dB SPL.

Table 2.2 shows the relationship between pressure measured and dB SPL. You can solve the others for practice.

Be sure to notice that if the *measured* pressure is 0.0002 dyne/cm², then the intensity is 0 dB SPL. Whenever the measured value is equal to the base value of the scale, the result is zero. This does not mean the absence of sound because the decibel is a relative scale.

$$\text{dB SPL} = 20 \times \log \frac{0.0002}{0.0002}$$

$$20 \times \log 1$$

Remember that the log of 1 is 0. Therefore, $20 \times 0 = \boxed{0 \text{ dB SPL}}$ .

Table 2.2.   Relationship of measured pressure to decibels (in sound pressure level)

| Measured pressure | dB SPL |
|---|---|
| 0.0002 | 0 (minimum audible sound) |
| 0.002 | 20 |
| 0.02 | 40 |
| 0.2 | 60 |
| 2.0 | 80 |
| 20.0 | 100 |
| 200.0 | 120 |
| 2000.0 | 140 (pain) |

Now look at Table 2.2; you should be able to see that every time you increase the intensity tenfold (one decimal place), there will be an increase of 20 dB SPL.

## SUMMARY

Intensity is the physical measure that is associated with the psychological sensation of loudness. The decibel is the standard unit for measuring intensity. In using the decibel, two important factors must be kept in mind. The first is that the dB is a unit based upon a logarithmic rather than a linear scale. Therefore, each successive dB unit represents a greater increase in intensity than the previous dB unit. Second, the dB scale is a relative scale which must have an arbitrary reference zero point. The decibel is actually a logarithmic ratio of the intensity measured to the reference intensity, which is normally 0.0002 dyne/cm². When this is the reference for our dB scale, we always add the suffix SPL to the dB value.

## GLOSSARY

*absolute scale*—A scale based upon a true zero point, or a point where that which is measured ceases to exist.

*decibel*—A relative unit of measurement which expresses the ratio between two values in a logarithmic form. The number of decibels (written dB) for sound pressure values may be calculated using the formula

$$N_{dB} = 20 \log (P_1/P_0)$$

where $P_1$ is the sound pressure that is measured and $P_0$ is a recognized reference point. Most often in audiology, the reference pressure is 0.0002 dyne/cm².

*dyne*—A unit of force. One dyne equals the force necessary to accelerate a mass of 1 gram to a velocity of 1 cm per second.

*linear scale*—A scale in which all the measurement units represent the same amount of change. For example, the distance on a ruler between 2 and 4 inches and 10 and 12 inches is exactly the same.

*logarithmic scale*—A scale in which each successive unit is larger than the one that precedes it. The decibel is a measurement unit that uses a logarithmic scale.

*relative scale*—A scale in which the zero point does not represent the absence of what is being measured. The scale value 0 is usually set, by consensus, to some point that has particular relevance. For example, 0° Celsius is arbitrarily set to the temperature at which water freezes, although temperature continues well below this value.

*sound pressure level*—Sound pressure level, in decibels, is 20 times the logarithmic ratio of the measured sound pressure to a reference sound pressure. Most often, the reference pressure is 0.0002 dyne/cm², which is considered to represent the lower limit of normal hearing. The reference pressure can also be stated in other physical terms, such as Newtons per square meter ($2 \times 10^{-5}$ N/m²), microbars ($2 \times 10^{-4}$ $\mu$bar), or micropascals (20 $\mu$Pa).

## SUGGESTED READING FOR FURTHER STUDY

Berlin, C. I. 1976. Programmed instruction in the decibel. In J. L. Northern (ed.), *Hearing Disorders*, Appendix. Little, Brown & Company, Boston. An excellent self-teacher on decibels.

## STUDY QUESTIONS

1. The reference point for the SPL scale in decibels is _____.
2. The decibel is a unit of _____.
3. _____ is created when force is applied over an area.
4. A scale in which all units are equivalent is referred to as a _____ scale.
5. A scale in which the zero point represents the absence of the measure is known as an _____ scale.
6. If you double the pressure, you will add _____ dB.
7. The logarithm of one is _____.
8. The loudest sound that the normal human ear can hear without pain is about _____ dB SPL.
9. The log of $10^6$ is _____.
10. An exponent is also known as a _____.

# PART II
## ANATOMY
## AND
## PHYSIOLOGY
## OF THE
## AUDITORY
## MECHANISM

# CHAPTER 3
## Overview
## of the Ear

The human auditory system can be divided into three main portions: the *conductive mechanism*, the *sensorineural mechanism*, and the *central mechanism* (Figure 3.1).

The primary function of the outermost portion, the conductive mechanism, is to bring the vibrational sound energy from outside the head to the inner portions of the ear so they can be used by the sensorineural mechanism. The conductive mechanism begins at the *pinna* or external ear. Although the pinna is highly visible on the side of the head, it is of minimal importance in hearing, and abnormalities of the pinna are primarily of cosmetic concern.

The pinna leads to the opening of a short, narrow tube called the *external auditory meatus* (*EAM*), or ear canal. The ear canal is terminated by a highly elastic membrane known as the *tympanic membrane*, or eardrum. Beyond the eardrum is a small air-filled space known as the *middle ear*. The middle ear contains three small bones, the *ossicles*, that bridge the tympanic membrane to the inner ear.

Since the sensory receptors of the ear are located in the inner ear, any portion of the sound that is lost crossing the conductive mechanism will not be heard. Therefore, the efficiency of the conductive mechanism in transporting the sound energy from the pinna to the inner ear is critical to the sensitivity of the auditory mechanism.

If an abnormality were to occur somewhere in the conductive mechanism which interfered with the normal flow of sound energy from the pinna through the middle ear, a hearing loss would occur. We refer to a hearing loss caused by an abnormality of the conductive mechanism as a *conductive hearing loss*. Perforations of the tympanic membrane and fluid filling the middle ear space are two examples of abnormalities that may cause a conductive hearing loss.

The *cochlea* is the sensory organ of hearing. It is a spiral-shaped organ that is responsible for converting the sound energy carried inward by the conductive mechanism into a neurological code that can be interpreted by the central auditory mechanism. This neurological code

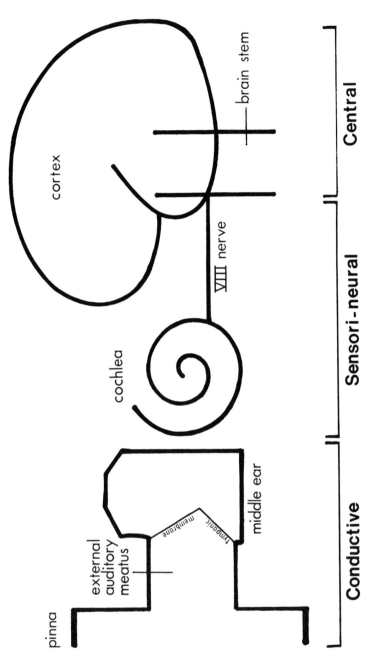

Figure 3.1.　Schematic of the auditory system.

Table 3.1.    Anatomical directions

| Name | Direction |
|------|-----------|
| Superior | Upward, above |
| Inferior | Downward, below |
| Medial | Toward the center or middle |
| Lateral | Toward the outside or periphery |
| Anterior | Toward the front |
| Posterior | Toward the back |

that now represents the auditory stimulus is carried by the *VIII cranial nerve* (the *auditory nerve*) to the central auditory mechanism. The cochlea and the VIII nerve are known jointly as the sensorineural portion of the auditory mechanism. Any hearing loss caused by dysfunction of the sensorineural mechanism is called a *sensorineural hearing loss.*

The central auditory mechanism is responsible for the recognition, interpretation, and integration of auditory information. The auditory message, after being encoded by the cochlea, passes through the brainstem on its way to the cortex. The auditory pathways through the brainstem and the auditory areas in the cortex are referred to as the *central auditory mechanism.* Damage to this portion of the mechanism may result in a *central hearing loss.* This type of loss causes inability to recognize, utilize, or understand sounds, rather than the loss of sensitivity that is characteristic of conductive or sensorineural losses. The term *peripheral* is sometimes used in opposition to *central*; therefore, the peripheral hearing mechanism refers to the whole of the conductive and sensorineural mechanisms.

As we continue with a more detailed study of the anatomy (structure) and physiology (function) of the ear, it will be necessary to describe relative locations of structures. The ease of this task will be greatly increased if the reader becomes familiar with the terms listed in Table 3.1.

The focus of our discussion of the structure of the ear is to provide the functional anatomy necessary to the understanding of the physiology and pathology of the auditory mechanism and to avoid minute detail. More detailed sources are suggested at the end of each of the chapters for further study.

First we will deal with the structure, function, and dysfunction of the conductive mechanism, and then, following the same organization, proceed to the sensorineural and central mechanisms.

**GLOSSARY**

*auditory nerve (VIII cranial nerve)*—The nerve that conveys neurological information from the inner ear structures to the central nervous system. It is also commonly referred to as the VIII cranial nerve. The auditory nerve is one portion of the sensorineural mechanism; the other portion is the cochlea.

*central auditory mechanism*—The various neurological pathways that exist from the brainstem to the auditory areas in the cerebral cortex.

*central hearing loss*—Occurs when there is some abnormality in the central auditory mechanism; that is, when an abnormal condition exists anywhere from the level of the brainstem to the auditory cortex.

*cochlea*—The spiral-shaped portion of the inner ear that contains the sensory organ of hearing. The cochlea is one portion of the sensorineural mechanism; the other portion is the auditory nerve (VIII nerve).

*conductive hearing loss*—Occurs when there is some abnormality in the conductive mechanism; that is, when an abnormal condition exists in the outer or middle ears.

*conductive mechanism*—The purpose of the ear's conductive mechanism is to first collect sound energy and then to change (transduce) this airborne energy into mechanical vibration so that it can be processed by the sensorineural mechanism. It is made up of the outer and middle ear.

*external auditory meatus* (*ear canal*)—The open channel from the concha to the tympanic membrane. The purpose of the external auditory meatus is to direct acoustic energy to the middle ear. The external auditory meatus is commonly referred to as the ear canal.

*inner ear*—The innermost. portion of the ear, which consists of the cochlea, the vestibular mechanism, and the auditory nerve (VIII cranial nerve). The purpose of the inner ear is to convert vibrational energy from the middle ear to neurological impulses which are sent to the central auditory system for interpretation.

*middle ear*—An air-filled space located in the temporal bone, which contains three small bones (the ossicles) and the eardrum. The purpose of the middle ear is to transfer sound energy from the outer ear to the inner ear.

*outer ear*—The outermost portion of the ear, which consists of the pinna and the external auditory meatus (ear canal). The purpose of the outer ear is to collect sound energy and deliver it to the middle ear.

*pinna*—The visible portion of the outer ear. It is composed of cartilage and characterized by a number of depressions. The pinna is also called the *auricle*.

*sensorineural hearing loss*—Occurs when there is some abnormality in the sensorineural mechanism; that is, when an abnormal condition exists in the cochlea or VIII nerve.

*sensorineural mechanism*—The cochlea and the auditory branch of the VIII cranial nerve. The purpose of the sensorineural mechanism is to receive the vibrational energy provided by the conductive mechanism, and convert (transduce) this energy into a neurological code so that it can be used by the central nervous system.

*tympanic membrane* (*eardrum*)—The membrane that separates the outer from middle ear. The tympanic membrane is composed of three distinct tissue layers; a skin layer that is continuous with the external auditory meatus, a middle fibrous layer, and a mucous layer that is continuous with the mucous lining of the middle ear.

**STUDY QUESTIONS**

1. The sensory organ of hearing is called the _____.
2. A hearing loss that results from damage to the outer or middle ear is called a _____ hearing loss.
3. The canal leading to the tympanic membrane is called the _____.
4. A hearing loss that is characterized by a loss of understanding rather than hearing sensitivity is called a _____.
5. The nerve for hearing is the _____ cranial nerve.

# CHAPTER 4
## The Structure of the Conductive Mechanism

### THE PINNA

The outermost portion of the conductive mechanism is known as the pinna or auricle. As we noted in the last chapter, the human pinna is primarily cosmetic and of questionable function. The pinna is constructed of skin and cartilage and is characterized by a variety of depressions, grooves, and ridges. The deepest depression leads directly to the external auditory meatus and is called the *concha*. The pinna varies somewhat in appearance from individual to individual, and tends to become larger and harder with age. The major landmarks of the pinna are shown in Figure 4.1.

### THE EXTERNAL AUDITORY MEATUS

The external auditory meatus begins at the concha and travels 25 mm to 35 mm (about 1 to 1¼ inches) to the tympanic membrane, which separates the external auditory meatus from the middle ear. It is mildly S shaped, bending upward toward the tympanic membrane. The lateral third of the ear canal is composed of cartilage while the medial or inner two-thirds is bony (Figure 4.2). The entire canal is lined with a thin layer of skin.

Since the cartilaginous portion is flexible, it is possible to straighten out the ear canal by pulling the pinna upward and backward; now the tympanic membrane can be observed with a special lighted magnifying instrument called an *otoscope* (Figure 4.3).

The skin of the cartilaginous portion contains two sets of glands which combine to produce a bitter, sticky, yellow substance known as *cerumen*, or ear wax. The cartilaginous portion of the ear canal also contains a number of hair follicles. The cerumen and hairs are thought to discourage the passage of foreign objects, such as insects, to the tympanic membrane.

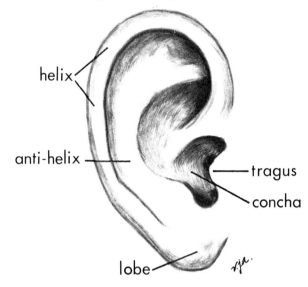

helix

anti-helix

tragus

concha

lobe

Figure 4.1.    The pinna.

## THE TYMPANIC MEMBRANE

The tympanic membrane or eardrum is a thin and highly elastic membrane that separates the ear canal from the middle ear. The normal tympanic membrane is pearly gray in color and varies from almost transparent to barely translucent.

The eardrum is composed of three layers. The outer layer is constructed of, and is continuous with, the layer of skin that lines the external auditory meatus. The inside layer is continuous with the mucous membrane lining of the middle ear. The middle layer, which is sandwiched between the skin and mucous layers, is fibrous in construction and accounts for the toughness and elasticity of the tympanic membrane.

The fibrous layer consists of radial fibers, which originate near the center of the tympanic membrane and spread toward the periphery, and circular fibers, which ring the tympanic membrane. The radial fibers are similar to spokes in a wheel; they are dense in the center and more sparse toward the periphery. The circular fibers, on the other hand, are sparse near the center and more numerous toward the periphery.

The outer edge of the tympanic membrane is a relatively thick ring of interwoven fibers and cartilage, which fits tightly into a groove in the bony wall of the external auditory meatus called the *tympanic sulcus*. This causes the eardrum to be firmly held to the ear canal. The groove is incomplete on the superior edge of the tympanic membrane, where the

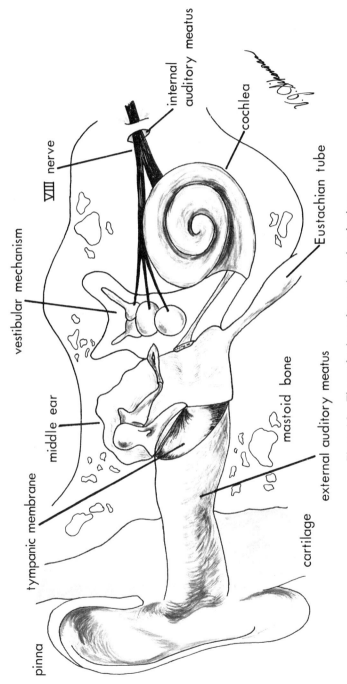

internal auditory meatus

cochlea

VIII nerve

Eustachian tube

vestibular mechanism

middle ear

mastoid bone

external auditory meatus

tympanic membrane

cartilage

pinna

Figure 4.2.    The conductive and sensorineural mechanisms.

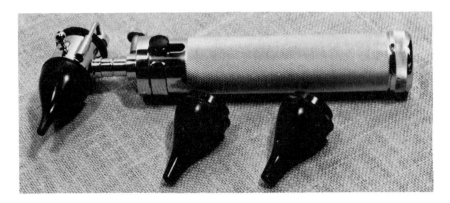

Figure 4.3.    An otoscope.

drum is held more loosely by a series of ligaments. The missing piece of bone on the superior side of the tympanic sulcus is called the *notch of Rivinus*. A small triangular area of the tympanic membrane, bound superiorly by the notch of Rivinus, is rather flaccid and is referred to as the *pars flaccida* or *Shrapnell's membrane*. In comparison, the remainder of the drum is held tautly, and is referred to as the *pars tensa*.

The *malleus*, the lateral bone of the ossicular chain, is firmly attached to the fibrous layer of the tympanic membrane. The malleus is positioned so that the tympanic membrane is pulled inward toward the middle ear. Therefore the shape of the eardrum is concave when viewed from the ear canal; the center point of the tympanic membrane, which is the tip of the conical shape, is called the *umbo* (Figures 4.4 and 4.5).

Just beyond the tympanic membrane is a small, roughly cube-shaped, air-filled space called the middle ear, or *tympanic cavity*. The adult middle ear is about ½ inch high and wide and about ¼ inch in depth (lateral to medial) (Figure 4.5).

The tympanic cavity is divided into two areas known as the *tympanic cavity proper* and the *epitympanic recess* or *attic*. The tympanic cavity proper is in the direct line of vision of the tympanic membrane. Above this, extending from the upper border of the tympanic membrane to the roof of the middle ear, is the attic.

As with any cube, there are six sides or walls. The superior wall, or roof, and the inferior wall, or floor, are thin shelves of bone and are of little consequence from the viewpoint of auditory functioning. Suffice it to say, however, that the superior wall separates the middle ear from the brain and the inferior wall separates the middle ear from the jugular vein.

The lateral wall of the middle ear is primarily formed by the tympanic membrane, with a section of bone superior to it in the attic portion of the middle ear.

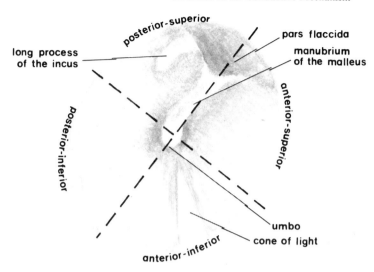

Figure 4.4.    Schematic of the right tympanic membrane showing its division into four quadrants.

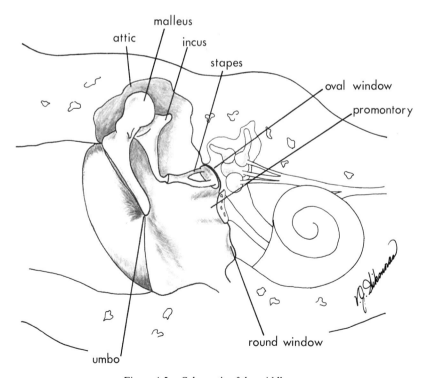

Figure 4.5.    Schematic of the middle ear.

## MEDIAL WALL

The medial wall of the middle ear contains four important structures. Two of these are openings or windows through the medial wall into the inner ear or labyrinth. The larger of the two is the *oval window*, and lying inferior and slightly anterior to it is the smaller *round window*. The round window is partially hidden in a cone-shaped depression called the *niche* of the round window; the window itself is covered by a thin membrane which is known as the *internal tympanic membrane*.

There is a bump or protrusion between the two windows called the *promontory*. This projection into the middle ear allows extra room on the other side of the wall for the first turn of the cochlea, which is part of the inner ear.

Just superior to the oval window is a small bony ridge which hides the VII cranial (facial) nerve as it passes through the middle ear. Figure 4.6 is a schematic of the medial wall of the middle ear. In addition to the VII nerve, there is also one other important nonauditory structure in the middle ear: the *chorda tympani*. This is a small branch of the facial nerve that passes through the middle ear itself, between the ossicles, and serves to carry information about taste from the anterior portion of the tongue to the central nervous system. The location of the chorda tympani sometimes causes it to interfere with middle ear surgery.

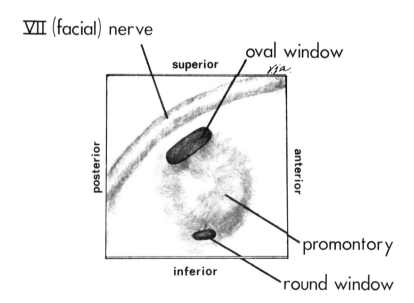

Figure 4.6.    Schematic of the medial wall of the middle ear.

## POSTERIOR WALL

The posterior wall contains one important landmark, a prominence parallel in height to the oval window, called the *pyramidal eminence*. It is hollow and contains the stapedius muscle, the smallest muscle in the human body, and one of the two muscles of the middle ear. There is a pinhole opening at the tip of the pyramidal eminence that allows the stapedius muscle tendon to emerge into the middle ear.

### ANTERIOR WALL

The anterior wall of the middle ear contains two significant landmarks. Buried in a small cavity in the wall is the second middle ear muscle, the *tensor tympani*. Inferior to the tensor tympani, separated by a thin shelf of bone, is the internal opening (or orifice) of the *Eustachian tube*. The adult Eustachian tube is about 35 mm long and connects the middle ear to an area in the back of the nose and throat called the nasopharynx. There are three muscles on the nasopharynx side of the tube that serve to open it upon yawning, swallowing, and sneezing. The Eustachian tube remains in a closed position at other times.

The Eustachian tube serves three main functions. One is to equalize air pressure on both sides of the tympanic membrane. If the pressure in the external auditory meatus is either increased or decreased, as is common in an airplane, the only way to equalize the pressure is by opening the Eustachian tube. The tube also allows for the air supply that is essential to the metabolism of the tissues of the middle ear. Last, the drainage of middle ear secretions into the nasopharynx is accomplished through the Eustachian tube.

A child's Eustachian tube is significantly shorter, wider, and straighter than an adult's, and therefore it is much more susceptible to disruption of normal functioning as well as to the spread of infection from the nose and throat to the middle ear.

### THE OSSICLES

A chain of three small bones crosses from the lateral wall to the medial wall of the middle ear: the malleus, the incus, and the stapes (pronounced "stāpēz"). Jointly the bones are known as the *ossicles*, or *ossicular chain*.

The ossicles are shown individually and labeled in Figure 4.7. The long arm or *manubrium* of the malleus is firmly attached to the tympanic membrane. The head of the malleus articulates or joins with the incus at the *incudomalleolar joint;* this is a *double saddle-type joint* that holds these two ossicles together tightly. At normal intensity levels, the malleus and incus are thought to operate as a single unit.

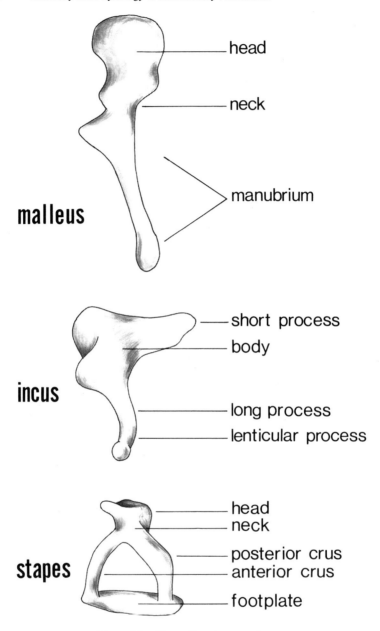

Figure 4.7.    The malleus, incus, and stapes.

The long process of the incus bends sharply at the inferior side to form the *lenticular process*, which articulates with the head of the stapes. This *incudostapedial joint* is a *ball and socket-type joint*, and the junction is significantly more flexible than the incudomalleolar joint; it is subject to separation from some head traumas (see Figure 4.8). The *footplate* of the stapes sits in the oval window and is held in place by the *annular ligament*. The attachment of the annular ligament is discussed in more detail in the next chapter when the motion of the stapes is discussed.

The ossicles are suspended from the roof of the attic by a series of ligaments. The ossicular chain (Figure 4.9) is covered with the same

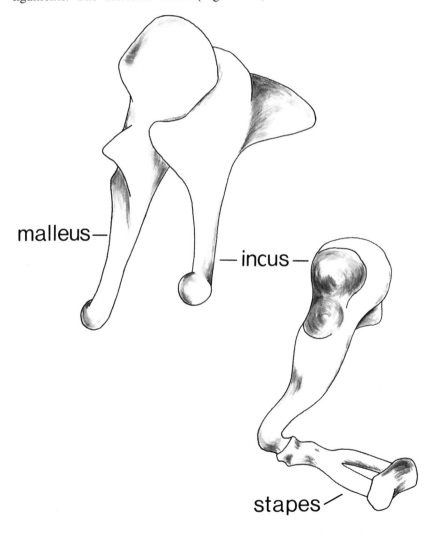

malleus—

—incus—

stapes

Figure 4.8.    The junction of the malleus and incus and of the incus and stapes.

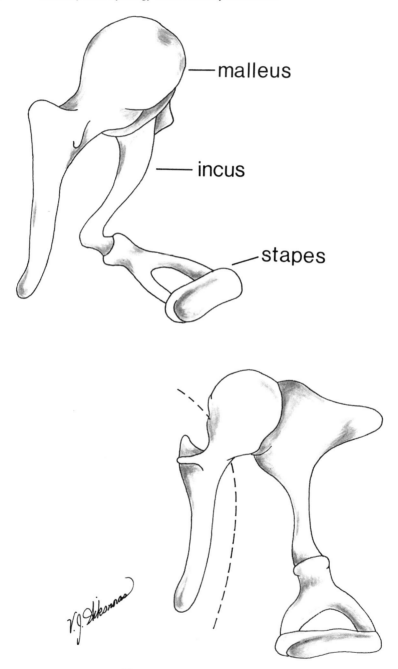

Figure 4.9.    The ossicular chain.

mucous membrane lining that covers the middle ear walls and forms the inside layer of the tympanic membrane.

## THE MIDDLE EAR MUSCLES

As we noted earlier, there are two small muscles in the middle ear. The stapedius muscle lies in the posterior wall of the middle ear; the stapedius tendon connects the muscle to the neck of the stapes. When the muscle contracts, the stapes is moved in a posterior direction. The stapedius muscle is innervated by a branch of the facial or VII cranial nerve.

The tensor tympani muscle lies in the anterior wall of the middle ear; its tendon connects the muscle to the manubrium of the malleus near the neck.

The tensor tympani is innervated by a branch of the V cranial (trigeminal) nerve; its innervation is complex and may well be served by other cranial nerves as well as the trigeminal. Upon contraction of the muscle it pulls essentially in an opposite direction to the stapedius muscle and serves to stiffen the tympanic membrane.

Sound energy passes through the external auditory meatus and is collected by the tympanic membrane. It is then passed through the middle ear through the ossicular chain to the inner ear. The next chapter deals with the physiology or function of the conductive mechanism, and those abnormalities of the conductive mechanism that can cause a loss of hearing.

## GLOSSARY

*annular ligament*—A ring of elastic fibers that encircles the stapes footplate, holding the stapes in the oval window.

*cerumen*—A wax-like secretion produced by specialized glands in the external auditory meatus. Cerumen is commonly referred to as ear wax.

*chorda tympani*—A branch of the facial (VII cranial) nerve that passes through the middle ear. It carries information about taste from the front portion of the tongue to the central nervous system.

*concha*—The hollowed-out portion of the pinna that adjoins the external ear canal.

*Eustachian tube (auditory tube)*—A channel that joins the tympanic cavity to the nasopharynx. Its purpose is to equalize the air pressure in the tympanic cavity to the outside pressure, to allow air into the middle ear, and to remove secretions from the tympanic cavity.

*incus*—The middlemost bone in the ossicular chain. It joins the malleus to the stapes.

*malleus*—One of the three middle ear ossicles. It is the most lateral of the ossicles, and is partially embedded in the tympanic membrane.

*manubrium*—The long arm or process of the malleus which is embedded in the fibrous layer of the tympanic membrane.

*notch of Rivinus*—Also called the *tympanic notch*. It is formed by the gap in the tympanic sulcus. The notch is occupied by the highest portion of the eardrum, the *pars flaccida*. (See *tympanic sulcus*.)

*otoscope*—An instrument consisting of a light source and a magnifying lens, which is designed to observe the ear canal and the tympanic membrane.

*pars flaccida* (*Shrapnell's membrane*)—The small triangular-shaped portion of the upper eardrum. This area of the eardrum is quite thin and flaccid.

*pars tensa*—The entire eardrum, except for the small triangular-shaped area known as the *pars flaccida*.

*pyramidal eminence*—A small, bony projection from the posterior wall of the tympanic cavity from which the tendon of the stapedius muscle emerges.

*stapedius muscle*—One of the two tiny muscles of the middle ear. It arises from the posterior wall of the middle ear and its tendon is attached to the stapes. It is innervated by the VII cranial (facial) nerve.

*stapes*—The smallest and innermost bone in the ossicular chain. It is attached on one side to the incus and on the other side fits into the oval window.

*tensor tympani muscle*—One of the two tiny muscles found in the middle ear. It arises from the anterior wall and its tendon is attached to the malleus. It is innervated by the V (trigeminal) nerve.

*tympanic cavity*—The cavity of the middle ear. The cavity is roughly cube shaped and lined with mucous membrane. It contains the ossicular chain, the middle ear muscles, and the oval and round windows, among other structures. The tympanic cavity communicates with the nasopharynx through the Eustachian tube. It is also referred to as the middle ear.

*tympanic sulcus*—The groove in the bony portion of the external auditory meatus in which the tympanic membrane is attached.

## SUGGESTED READING FOR FURTHER STUDY

Zemlin, W. R. 1968. *Speech and Hearing Science: Anatomy and Physiology.* Prentice-Hall, Englewood Cliffs, N.J.
A detailed account of the anatomy.

**STUDY QUESTIONS**

1. The _____ is composed of the pinna and the external auditory meatus.
2. A lighted instrument used to examine the tympanic membrane is called an _____.
3. The eardrum is composed of two main parts: the _____ and the _____.
4. The middle layer of the tympanic membrane is composed of _____ and _____ fibers.
5. The ossicle that fits in the oval window is the _____.
6. The ossicle that is attached to the tympanic membrane is the _____.
7. The middle ear is connected to the nasopharynx by the _____.
8. The two muscles of the middle ear are the _____ and _____.
9. The bulge on the medial wall of the middle ear is called the _____.
10. The portion of the tympanic cavity above the eardrum is called the _____.

# CHAPTER 5

# The Function and Dysfunction of the Conductive Mechanism

As we have already mentioned, the primary function of the middle ear is to transfer acoustic energy from the pinna to the cochlea in the inner ear. In this chapter we will study this process in detail.

## OVERVIEW

Sound energy passes through the external auditory meatus and strikes the cone-shaped tympanic membrane. The sound wave causes the membrane to vibrate. This mechanical energy of the tympanic membrane vibrations is then transferred to the malleus, which is firmly attached to the tympanic membrane. This anatomical arrangement of the eardrum and the malleus allows an efficient transfer of energy and also serves to maintain the tense, cone shape of the tympanic membrane.

The malleus and incus normally act as a unit, and vibrate in correspondence with the motions of the tympanic membrane. The incus passes the energy along to the stapes, which is attached to the oval window by the *annular ligament*. The stapes footplate moves in and out as it is rocked by the incus; the mechanical energy is transferred to the inner ear through the oval window opening.

## THE MIDDLE EAR TRANSFORMER

### Impedance

The footplate of the stapes pushes into a water-like fluid on the other side of the oval window, called *perilymph*. This fluid, like all fluids, has a very high resistance to the flow of energy. The resistance to the flow of energy by a medium is known as *impedance*. Mediums that have a low resistance to such energy flow, such as air, are called *low impedance mediums*. When sound reaches a low impedance medium, most of the energy passes into the medium and very little is reflected away. Conversely, when sound reaches a very high impedance medium, little is absorbed into the medium and the majority is reflected away.

As Figure 5.1 illustrates, when sound has to flow from a low impedance medium (air in this case) to a high impedance medium (water), a great deal of energy will be reflected away and only a small amount will successfully be transferred.

The impedance of any medium is determined by the mass, stiffness, and friction of the medium. An increase in any of these three factors will reduce the flow of sound into a medium, and therefore increase the amount of reflected sound. Thus, if we cover existing walls of an average room with steel plates or lead sheeting, the sound insulation will be improved because more sound energy will be reflected away from the room.

**Impedance Mismatch**

The normal middle ear is very low in impedance. Some minimal impedance does exist because of such factors as the mass of the ossicles and tympanic membrane, the stiffness and friction of the ossicular joints, and the stiffness of the ossicular chain itself due to the outward pressure of the perilymph.

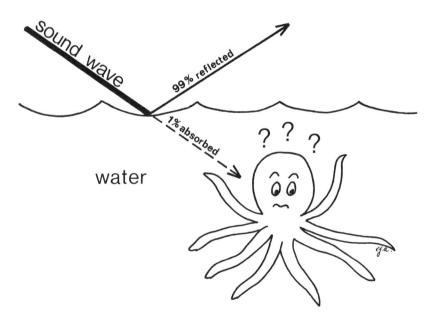

Figure 5.1.   Sound transfer from air to water.

The perilymph in the inner ear, on the other hand, is very high in impedance. When the transfer of sound is made from the low impedance of the middle ear to the high impedance of the perilymph, a great deal of energy must be lost. In this case, approximately 30 dB of sound will be reflected away from the inner ear and therefore lost to the auditory mechanism. If this were not compensated for in some manner, the amazing sensitivity of the hearing mechanism would not be possible. Considering the crucial alerting and protective function of the hearing sense, this could have had major effects on the development of the human species.

## Middle Ear Transformer

One critical function of the middle ear is to compensate for this potential 30-dB loss of hearing due to the impedance mismatch between the middle ear and the perilymph of the inner ear. There are two actions of the middle ear designed to accomplish this. One is called the *condensation effect* and the other is the *lever action* of the malleus and the incus.

**The Condensation Effect**  Sound is collected and transferred onward by the portion of the tympanic membrane known as the pars tensa, or the *effective area of the tympanic membrane*. This energy is delivered through the ossicular chain to the much smaller area of the stapes footplate. The effective area of the eardrum is about 13 times larger than the stapes footplate.

Basic physics tells us that pressure, such as sound pressure, is determined by a force being distributed over an area:

$$\text{Pressure} = \frac{\text{Force}}{\text{Area}}$$

If the force is held constant, but the area is reduced, then an increase in pressure will result.

When the sound pressure collected by the effective area of the tympanic membrane is condensed to the 13-times-smaller stapes footplate, such an amplification of pressure occurs. When measured in decibels, an increase of approximately 23 dB occurs because of the reduction in area (Figure 5.2).

**Lever Action**  A simple lever, such as a common children's seesaw, can be used to obtain a significant mechanical advantage. If the two arms of the lever are equal in length, as in Figure 5.3, then no advantage will be seen. However, if the pivot (fulcrum) of the seesaw is adjusted so that the arms are unequal, as in Figure 5.4, a lighter person on side A (the long arm) will be able to lift a heavier person on side B. If A were twice as long as B, a lever ratio or mechanical amplification of 2:1 would result. Actually, arm A would be moving a greater distance than arm B in order to create the increased upward pressure that lifts the heavier person on arm B (Figure 5.5).

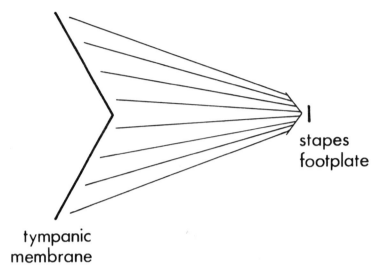

stapes
footplate

tympanic
membrane

Figure 5.2.    The condensation effect.

There is a second action of the middle ear that contributes to offsetting the impedance mismatch between the middle ear cavity and the fluid of the inner ear. The malleus and the incus form a lever which results in a reduction of movement from the malleus to the incus of about 1.3 to 1. This advantageous lever ratio results in a sound amplification of approximately 2 dB as sound crosses the ossicular chain.

In summary, the middle ear provides an efficient solution to the problem of the impedance mismatch. After the acoustic energy is collected by the tympanic membrane and changed into mechanical energy, approximately 23 dB of amplification are added by the condensation of energy at the footplate of the stapes from the much larger tympanic membrane, and about 2 dB are contributed by the lever advantage of the ossicular chain. Therefore, a total of 25 dB are added to make up for the 30-dB loss that occurs when energy is reflected away from the perilymph.

Obviously, the 25 dB do not completely offset the 30-dB energy loss. Two points of view seem to exist on this. Some writers believe that the middle ear *transformer action* is not quite perfect and recovers only

A                    B

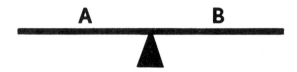

Figure 5.3.    The lever with two equal arms.

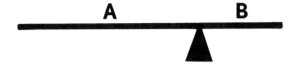

Figure 5.4.    A lever with unequal arms.

about 25 dB, which is sufficient to largely compensate for the loss of hearing caused by the impedance mismatch. Others believe that the system really compensates for essentially all of the 30 dB and that technical and experimental measurement error accounts for the missing 5 dB.

It should be noted that in an ear with a broken or absent ossicular chain, a loss as large as 50 dB to 60 dB is seen. However, this is due only in part to the 25- to 30-dB loss caused by the lack of a transformer action; several other factors, such as the energy loss resulting from sound not being directed at the oval window, must also be taken into account.

## ACTION OF THE MIDDLE EAR MUSCLES

### Acoustic Reflex

The two muscles of the middle ear, the stapedius and the tensor tympani, fire as part of a reflex action. Both muscles contract bilaterally, regardless of which ear is stimulated.

The stapedius muscle fires at intensities of about 60 dB above hearing threshold when a noise stimulus is used to elicit the reflex; approximately 20 dB more are needed if a pure tone stimulus is employed.

The tensor tympani appears to contract at greater intensities than the stapedius. It also is known to respond to a variety of tactile stimuli and as part of the gross startle response.

When contracted, the stapedius muscle produces a significant increase in the impedance of the middle ear. This is caused primarily by

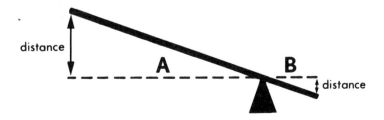

Figure 5.5.    Relation of distance moved to arm length in a lever.

an increase in the stiffness of the ossicular chain, which is caused by the posterior pull of the stapedius tendon. As we know, an increase in middle ear impedance will cause a reduction in the flow of sound to the inner ear. This transmission loss, which occurs only at high intensities, serves to protect the inner ear from the trauma of loud sounds.

In addition to the increased stiffness of the ossicular chain, the piston-like movement of the stapes footplate that occurs for low intensity and moderate intensity sounds is modified. Because the annular ligament is thicker at the posterior and inferior borders of the footplate, there is more freedom of movement at the anterior border than at the posterior border. At high intensities, because of the structure of the annular ligament, the footplate moves more like a door with its hinges at the posterior border than like a piston. This acts to dampen the energy transmitted to the perilymph.

Although it is known that a contraction of the tensor tympani muscle pulls the tympanic membrane inward, the effect on the impedance of the middle ear, and therefore on sound transmission to the inner ear, is still controversial. A number of writers feel that the contraction of the tensor tympani is ineffective in increasing the impedance of the human ear, and therefore the muscle is inconsequential as part of the protective mechanism.

### Effect on Threshold

The middle ear muscle or acoustic reflex is known to attenuate sound about 12 dB to 14 dB in the lower frequencies; little effect is seen above 1000 Hz. Although some protection is undoubtedly afforded the inner ear against loud sounds, the amount of transmission loss is certainly not adequate to the task for exposures to sounds of great intensity. Furthermore, the attenuation effect of the acoustic reflex is known to have a latency of 60 milliseconds to 120 milliseconds. This would suggest that any damage from instantaneous sounds, such as gunshots, would not be prevented by the reflex—in essence, closing the barn door after the horse has exited.

## DISORDERS OF THE CONDUCTIVE MECHANISM

### The Pinna

As we have noted before, malformations of the pinna have little effect on hearing, and any such abnormalities are primarily the concern of a plastic surgeon.

### The External Auditory Meatus

A closed external auditory meatus is known as an *atresia*. Ear canal atresias are sometimes associated with other congenital abnormalities of the tympanic membrane and middle ear structures. Such canal closures cause conductive hearing losses as large as 60 dB. Although it is sometimes possible to correct a canal atresia with surgery, complications such as associated middle ear malformations often make this type of surgery unsuccessful.

If cerumen collects and hardens in the external auditory meatus (*impacted cerumen*) in sufficient quantity to completely block the flow of sound, a hearing loss will result. This type of loss is temporary, with normal hearing returning when the blockage is removed.

When the skin of the external auditory meatus becomes inflamed and infected, the condition is referred to as *external otitis;* this does not normally produce a hearing loss unless the swelling is sufficient to completely close the external auditory meatus. Patients usually complain of itching and pain, both of which may become rather severe. The otologist normally treats the condition with antibiotic eardrops and may also employ an anti-inflammatory steroid drug. If the swelling is severe, care must be taken to ensure that the drops are able to reach the infected areas of the ear canal. Sometimes it is necessary to put a cotton wick in the ear canal and saturate the wick with an antibiotic solution.

### The Tympanic Membrane

Perforations of the tympanic membrane produce a hearing loss that varies greatly depending on the size and exact location of the perforation. Small, regular perforations tend to heal spontaneously, while larger or irregular perforations are more likely to form scar tissue. It is sometimes necessary to surgically repair the tympanic membrane using a grafting technique; this operation is known as *myringoplasty.*

### Serous Otitis Media

For a variety of reasons, the normal function of the Eustachian tube may be interrupted. Most commonly, the culprit is a swelling of the Eustachian tube due to allergies, an inflammation of the tube secondary to a nose or throat infection, or a blockage of the nasopharynx orifice of the Eustachian tube by enlarged adenoids. This can prevent the opening of the tube during yawning and swallowing, and air no longer flows into the middle ear.

The air in the middle ear is absorbed by the mucous membrane causing the formation of a partial vacuum, sometimes referred to as negative middle ear pressure. The tympanic membrane is retracted, or pulled inward, by the pressure imbalance, and sometimes fluid is secreted from the mucous membrane into the middle ear cavity. The presence of this noninfected fluid and negative middle ear pressure, all related to Eustachian tube malfunction, is known as *serous otitis media* or nonsuppurative otitis media.

An otologist will normally prescribe a decongestant and antihistamine to dry up the fluid and open the Eustachian tube. If the fluid continues to accumulate, the otologist may find it necessary to surgically open the tympanic membrane in order to drain the fluid. Sometimes a small tube is inserted into the tympanic membrane to temporarily act in place of the Eustachian tube, allowing for ventilation of the middle ear and drainage of the fluid, until normal Eustachian tube function can be restored. This surgical procedure is known as *myringotomy*.

At times, instead of the thin, watery fluid of serous otitis media, the effusion is a thick, dense noninfected material. This is referred to as *mucous otitis media* or "glue ear." The successful treatment of mucous otitis media is often difficult, and, if the effusion remains too long, a series of middle ear adhesions may form which can restrict the movement of the ossicles.

## Purulent Otitis Media

If an infection invades the middle ear, instead of a clear fluid, the middle ear fills with pus. The primary source of these bacteria is the nasopharynx, although perforation of the tympanic membrane may also allow the infection to enter the middle ear. This condition is often accompanied by intense pain. This infection of the middle ear is known as *purulent otitis media* or suppurative otitis media.

In its early stages, this is referred to as acute purulent otitis media, but if it continues over a period of several months, particularly if a tympanic membrane perforation persists, it is referred to as *chronic otitis media*.

The otologist employs antibiotic therapy to counteract purulent otitis media. Sometimes direct removal of the pus with a myringotomy in addition to drug therapy is the appropriate course of treatment. If the infection process spreads to the mastoid bone it is referred to as *mastoiditis*. If antibiotics are not effective in eliminating the infection, a surgical procedure called a *mastoidectomy* may be necessary in order to remove the infected bone tissue.

## Otosclerosis

*Otosclerosis* begins as a soft, spongy growth of new bone in the middle ear that hardens with time. Although otosclerotic growth can occur anywhere in the middle ear, it normally causes a hearing loss only when it forms on or around the stapes footplate. As the otosclerotic growth accumulates and hardens, the mobility of the stapes diminishes, and therefore sound is not transmitted as efficiently to the inner ear. Gradually, the footplate becomes totally fixated in the oval window.

Otosclerosis begins in youth and is a slowly progressive disease; its associated hearing loss is usually first noted in the late teens to early 30s. It tends to run in families, appears predominantly in Caucasians, and is about twice as common in women as in men.

The disease causes no pain or other physical discomforts aside from the hearing loss and a ringing, humming, or buzzing noise in the ear called tinnitus. Otosclerosis may affect one or both ears.

There is no medical treatment know for otosclerosis. A surgical technique called *stapedectomy* is commonly used to improve hearing. This involves the removal of the fixated stapes and its replacement with a prosthesis. Stapedectomy, in the hands of a skilled otologist, is a highly successful procedure with minimal associated risk.

**Other Middle Ear Disorders**

We have by no means exhausted the list of all possible pathological conditions of the conductive mechanism. A few others that are important to the audiologist are mentioned briefly.

A *cholesteatoma* is a cyst of the middle ear that can be extremely dangerous. As it becomes larger, the cholesteatoma usually grows rapidly and occupies the middle ear space, often destroying bone and other tissue. The primary treatment is surgical removal.

Head trauma can result in a separation of an ossicular joint or the fracture of an ossicle; this is known as an *ossicular discontinuity*. A variety of tumors that can be either benign or malignant may also form in the tympanic cavity. Chronic purulent otitis media and cholesteatomas can result in sufficient damage to the middle ear to require reconstructive surgery of the middle ear. This reconstructive operation is called a *tympanoplasty*.

Several basic texts in audiology and otology are recommended at the end of this chapter for those who wish to further explore the pathology and hearing losses of the conductive mechanism.

**GLOSSARY**

*atresia*—In medicine, associated with the closure of a normal opening. In the ear, an atresia would be associated with a closed external auditory meatus.

*cholesteatoma*—A cyst which typically grows from the upper portion of the tympanic membrane. A pouch is formed, into which the dead skin that lines the pouch sheds. As more skin is shed into the pouch, the cholesteatoma grows. The effect is that of a foreign object within the middle ear cavity. This may lead to erosion of the ossicles, the formation of pus, and a discharge from the ear.

*chronic otitis media*—Occurs when infection persists in the middle ear cavity for a prolonged time period. The ear will often discharge pus, which has a foul odor.

*condensation effect*—The condensation effect refers to one aspect of the transformer action of the middle ear. Sound is collected over a relatively large area (the eardrum) and is transferred to an area 13 times smaller—the stapes footplate. This, in effect, causes a pressure increase at the oval window, since the original force has remained unchanged, but the area has been reduced. This "condensation" of energy accounts for a considerable mechanical advantage of the middle ear (about 23 dB).

*external otitis* ("*swimmer's ear*")—Occurs when changes in the skin that lines the external auditory meatus permit the growth of bacteria or fungi. When this occurs there is considerable swelling of the canal walls. Hearing loss occurs only when the ear canal is completely closed.

*impacted cerumen*—A common cause of conductive hearing loss due to the blocking of the ear canal with cerumen.

*lever action*—The mechanical advantage that is gained through the combined effect of the malleus and the incus. This accounts for about 2 dB of the total 25 dB of amplification provided by the middle ear system.

*mastoidectomy*—A surgical operation that aims to remove diseased mastoid air cells. There are several forms of mastoidectomies, each with a different purpose.

*mastoiditis*—An inflammation of the mastoid air cells.

*mucous otitis media*—Occurs when the fluid present within the tympanic cavity is thickened. The thickened fluid is not infected. (See *serous otitis media*.)

*myringoplasty*—An operation designed to repair a perforation of the tympanic membrane.

*myringotomy*—A surgical incision of the eardrum to drain fluid or pus.

*nonsuppurative otitis media*—Those conditions in which fluid present within the middle ear cavity is noninfected. Both *serous otitis media* and *mucous otitis media* fall into this category.

*ossicular discontinuity*—Occurs whenever the ossicular chain is interrupted. The cause may be head trauma, fracture, or disease.

*otosclerosis*—A condition in which conductive hearing loss occurs, usually through a gradual fixation of the stapes in the oval window. Although the actual cause is unknown, a pathological condition occurs such that new bony growth is laid down around the stapes footplate. This, of course, impedes vibration of the stapes with a resulting conductive hearing loss.

*purulent otitis media*—See *suppurative otitis media.*

*serous otitis media*—A common cause of conductive loss. It may arise as the result of a head cold, allergies, enlarged adenoids, or other conditions that impair Eustachian tube function. The condition is characterized by the accumulation of clear, thin fluid within the middle ear cavity, which serves to impair sound conduction. Serous otitis media is also referred to as *nonsuppurative otitis media.*

*stapedectomy*—A surgical procedure to improve hearing in cases of otosclerosis. In this operation, the immobile stapes is first removed and is then replaced by a prosthesis. (See *otosclerosis.*)

*suppurative otitis media*—A condition in which fluid is present in the middle ear and the fluid has become infected (pus formation). This condition is also known as *purulent otitis media.*

*transformer action*—The biological amplification process in the middle ear that allows the efficient transfer of energy from the low impedance middle ear to the high impedance perilymph. The transformer action is made up of the condensation effect and the lever action.

*tympanoplasty*—A surgical procedure that aims to reconstruct the middle ear's conductive function. One form of tympanoplasty involves grafting various types of tissue to replace or repair a diseased or perforated eardrum.

## SUGGESTED READINGS FOR FURTHER STUDY

Davis, H., and S. R. Silverman. 1978. *Hearing and Deafness*, Chapters 4 and 6. 4th Ed. Holt, Rinehart & Winston, New York.
Excellent summary of diseases of the conductive mechanism.
Derlacki, E. L. 1976. Otosclerosis. In J. L. Northern (ed.), *Hearing Disorders*, Chapter 11. Little, Brown & Company, Boston.
Good discussion.
Martin, F. N. 1975. *Introduction to Audiology*, Chapters 6 and 7. Prentice-Hall, Englewood Cliffs, N.J.
Good introduction for the audiology student.
Payne, E. E., and M. M. Paparella. 1976. Otitis media. In J. L. Northern (ed.), *Hearing Disorders*, Chapter 10. Little, Brown & Company, Boston.
Good discussion.

**STUDY QUESTIONS**

1. The resistance to the flow of sound energy in a medium is _____ .

2. The impedance of a medium is determined by its _____, _____, and _____.

3. The amplification of pressure due to the reduction of area from the tympanic membrane to the stapes footplate is known as the _____.

4. The mechanical advantage provided by the malleus and incus is called the _____.

5. An abnormal closure of the external auditory meatus is called an _____.

6. If the transformer action of the middle ear were absent, we would expect a loss of hearing of about _____.

7. A disease that produces a bony growth that immobilizes the stapes is called _____.

8. An operation to open the tympanic membrane to drain fluid is known as a _____.

9. The presence of a clear, noninfected fluid in the middle ear is referred to as _____.

10. Reconstructive surgery of the middle ear is known as _____.

# CHAPTER 6
# The Structure of the
# Sensorineural Mechanism

The two preceding chapters were concerned with the ear's conductive mechanism. We saw that the conductive mechanism is essentially a mechanical system. First, the external ear canal intercepts acoustic energy; then the acoustic energy is converted to mechanical energy through the middle ear structures. In this regard, the transformer action of the middle ear provides a very efficient energy transfer from the airborne sounds to the fluids of the inner ear. The stapes is, of course, the most medial portion of the middle ear system. It is attached to the oval window, which is the entry to the inner ear. In this chapter, we shall concern ourelves with the structure of the inner ear, or the sensorineural mechanism.

## THE LABYRINTH

The inner ear lies within a hollowed-out area in the temporal bone of the skull. The inner ear is part of a larger structure called the *labyrinth*. As the name implies, the inner ear area is not regular in shape, but rather complex. The labyrinth actually consists of two separate portions, one completely contained within the other. The first portion, the *osseous*, or *bony, labyrinth*, represents the actual hollowed-out portion of the temporal bone. The bony labyrinth can be further divided into a series of three separate irregularly shaped areas which communicate with each other (see Figure 6.1). The first area, the *semicircular canals*, is concerned primarily with our sense of equilibrium, or balance. There are three canals (superior, lateral, and posterior) which are all at right angles to one another. The second portion of the bony labyrinth is the *cochlea*. The cochlea contains the organ of hearing and is, therefore, of most concern to us. The cochlea resembles a snail shell in that it is formed by a canal that spirals 2¾ turns around a central core of bone called the *modiolus*. The third part of the osseous labyrinth is the *vestibule*. The vestibule is the central portion of the labyrinth into which the cochlea and semicircular canals open on either end. The oval window is located

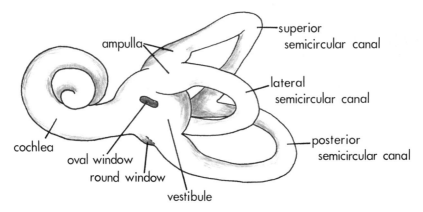

Figure 6.1.    The osseous labyrinth.

on the lateral wall of the vestibule. The entire bony labyrinth is filled with a fluid called *perilymph*.

We noted before that the labyrinth consists of two distinct parts, one housed within the other. The outer portion, as we have just seen, is the bony labyrinth. It is the hollowed-out portion of the temporal bone itself. The inner portion is called the *membranous labyrinth*. The membranous labyrinth consists of a series of communicating sacs and ducts which generally conform to the shape of the much larger bony labyrinth. Figure 6.2 shows the overall shape of the membranous labyrinth. Note the

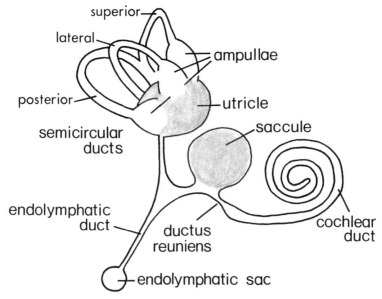

Figure 6.2.    The membranous labyrinth.

form of these structures relative to the overall form of the bony labyrinth as we saw in Figure 6.1. Although the membranous labyrinth is contained within the osseous labyrinth, the two contain different fluids. The bony labyrinth contains perilymph whereas the membranous labyrinth contains a liquid called *endolymph*.

## THE COCHLEA

The cochlea is the portion of the labyrinth directly concerned with hearing. We noted before that the cochlea is essentially a hollowed-out tube, which is coiled for nearly three turns around a central core of bone, the modiolus. The coiled nature of the cochlea makes it difficult for the introductory student to visualize its construction in three-dimensional space. As an aid in understanding cochlear construction, consider that the cochlea is simply a round tube or hose capable of being wound. By looking at this tube from various viewpoints, we will shortly see how they may be directly applied to the cochlea itself.

### Some Preliminaries

Figure 6.3 shows our illustrative tube from three viewpoints. Viewpoint *a* shows the tube stretched out. If we were to remove the near wall of the tube, we would be able to visualize the contents of the tube (if any) for the tube's entire length. This would be similar to viewing the contents through x-ray (see inset *a*). Viewpoint *b* shows another way to view the tube, looking into it from an end. If the tube were uniform in its dimensions for its entire length, then cutting it at any point (see inset *b*) would not alter viewpoint *b*. Viewpoint *c* requires a bit of imagination. Consider that our tube is wound almost three turns around a central post to form a coil. Each turn of the coil is a bit smaller than the one before. The first (basal) turn is the largest in diameter, and the third (apical) turn is the smallest in diameter. Next, imagine that we are somehow able to freeze the coil in place. If this were so, we would then be able to slice the whole coil down the center (see inset *c*). If we were to look into each of the halves of the bisected coil we would see five openings. Two of the openings would be from the first (basal) turn, two would be from the middle (medial) turn, and only one from the incomplete upper (apical) turn.

The remaining portion of this section concerns actual cochlear structure, and views the cochlea in much the same fashion as the bendable tube presented above. Figure 6.4 shows a schematic cochlea cut in half. Its resemblance to inset *c* of Figure 6.3 is obvious.

### Cochlear Structure

Consider some of the physical dimensions of the cochlea, which are astonishingly small. The spiral canal is only about 35 mm in length. In

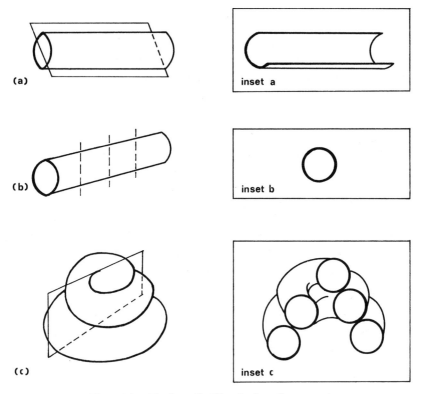

Figure 6.3.    Viewing a flexible tube from three aspects.

terms of height, it is only about 5 mm from the base to apex. The canal itself is about 8 mm to 9 mm across at the base, and smaller toward the apex.

Figure 6.5 shows a view of the cochlea in a highly schematic form. Notice that this particular view is similar to viewpoint *b* in Figure 6.3. In other words, we are viewing the cochlea from an end.

The first thing to be noted in the figure is that the cochlea is not a perfectly rounded structure. Notice that a thin shelf of bone protrudes into the canal from the central portion of the cochlea (the modiolus). This shelf of bone is called the *bony spiral lamina*. It extends down the cochlea for nearly its entire length. The only portion of the cochlea that is not partially separated by the lamina is in the region of the apex. A tough membrane, the *basilar membrane*, extends from the bony spiral lamina to the outer wall of the bony labyrinth. There it is held in place by the spiral ligament. The basilar membrane, in effect, separates the cochlea into two distinct channels for nearly its entire length. Figure 6.5 also shows another membrane to divide the cochlea. This is known as

*Reissner's membrane*, and it stretches diagonally from a fibrous membrane covering the bony spiral lamina, the *limbus*, to the outer wall of the bony labyrinth. There it is attached to a thickened portion of the spiral ligament. As is the case for the basilar membrane, Reissner's membrane continues along nearly the entire length of the cochlea. In the region of the apex, Reissner's membrane joins with the basilar membrane just before the end of the canal.

The cochlea, then, is divided into three separate channels. The uppermost channel is known as the *scala vestibuli*. It is formed by the bony labyrinth and Reissner's membrane. The lowermost channel is known as the *scala tympani*. It is formed by the bony labyrinth and the basilar membrane. Finally, a channel is formed between the basilar and Reissner's membranes. This channel is called the *scala media*, but it is also frequently referred to as the *cochlear duct* or *cochlear partition*.

We noted earlier that the cochlea, as does every other division of the inner ear, consists of bony and membranous portions. The latter are

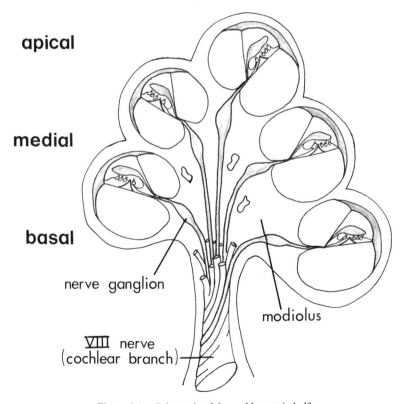

Figure 6.4.   Schematic of the cochlea cut in half.

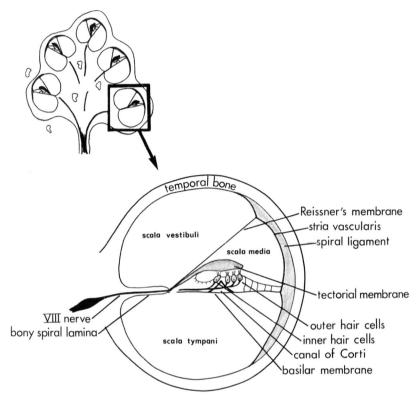

Figure 6.5.   A schematic view of one turn of the cochlea.

housed within the former. As far as the cochlea is concerned, the bony labyrinth consists of the scalae vestibuli and tympani. The membranous portion of the labyrinth is the scala media. We also noted that two different fluids fill the inner ear space, perilymph in the osseous labyrinth and endolymph in the membranous labyrinth. Therefore, the scalae vestibuli and tympani are filled with perilymph and the scala media with endolymph. A highly vascular layer of tissue, the *stria vascularis*, lines the inner surface of the spiral ligament. It is thought that the purpose of the stria vascularis is to secrete endolymph. Perilymph is thought to arise from the very fine tissue coverings that line the bony labyrinth.

At this point in our discussion it is sufficient to note only that the actual organ of hearing, the *organ of Corti*, is located within the scala media. This organ is a highly complex structure located on the upper side of the basilar membrane. Detailed study of the organ of Corti is reserved until later in this section.

Figure 6.6 is a highly schematic representation of the cochlea in its uncoiled state. It is therefore analogous to viewpoint *a* in Figure 6.3. For the sake of clarity, we have purposely distorted the size of the scala media relative to the overall size of the cochlea. In fact, the cross-sectional area of the scala media is about one-sixth that of the total cross-sectional area of the cochlea.

There are several relationships in Figure 6.6 that should solidify some of the material presented in the previous paragraphs. For one, we see here that the bony canal of the cochlea tapers as it progresses from the base to the apex. Notice too that the basilar and Reissner's membranes traverse nearly the entire length of the canal, joining each other a short distance from the end. This then forms the *helicotrema*, through which the perilymph in the scala vestibuli and scala tympani communicates.

The scala vestibuli and scala tympani are terminated by two separate structures at the basal end of the cochlea. The scala vestibuli is terminated by the oval window, which is closed by the stapes and annular ligament. The scala tympani is terminated by the round window membrane. To recall our middle ear anatomy for a moment, on the medial wall we find both the oval and round windows, the latter located just below the former. The promontory, the hump that separates the oval window from the round window, represents the basal turn of the cochlea.

Figure 6.6 shows us clearly that the scala media, formed superiorly by Reissner's membrane and inferiorly by the basilar membrane, is a system separate and apart from the other cochlear structures. This system, of course, is part of the membranous labyrinth. The endolymph at the basal end of the scala media communicates with the remainder of the membranous labyrinth through a small canal called the *ductus reuniens* (see Figure 6.2 for details).

Although Figure 6.6 gives a good side view of the cochlea in its uncoiled state, it does not show that, when viewed from above, the basilar membrane actually becomes wider as it progresses from the base to the apex even though the cochlea is becoming narrower. Its width is about 0.04 mm at the base and about 0.5 mm at the apex.

## THE ORGAN OF CORTI

We have alluded to the fact that the organ of hearing, the organ of Corti, is located within the scala media. This section is devoted to the structure of this organ. Discussion of the mechanism of stimulation is left to Chapter 7 on cochlear function.

Figure 6.7 shows a schematic view of the organ of Corti. Those structures of particular interest to us here are shaded. These shaded structures are used in the auditory receptive process. Those structures that are unshaded are essentially supportive in nature; that is, they serve to support the organ and maintain its shape.

Notice that the organ of Corti is divided into two sections by a triangular-shaped structure known as the *tunnel of Corti*. The tunnel is formed by two rows of rods called the *rods of Corti*. Notice that on the inner side of the rods is a single row of hair cells called the *internal* or *inner hair cells*. Notice too that there are supportive cells which flank the inner hair cells on their inner side. On the outer side of the rods are three (and sometimes four) rows of *external* or *outer hair cells*. These hair cells are held up by various types of supporting cells. It should be emphasized here that both the inner and outer hair cells are the actual sensory receptor cells for the hearing process. Both the inner and outer hair cells are connected to nerve fibers which leave the cochlea through openings in the spiral lamina. Those nerve fibers that are attached to the outer hair cells pass across the tunnel of Corti.

If we look closely at both the inner and outer hair cells, we see small, hair-like projections at their tops. These projections are known as *cilia*. The hair cells actually derive their names from the presence of the cilia. The cilia are supported and held together to a certain extent by a

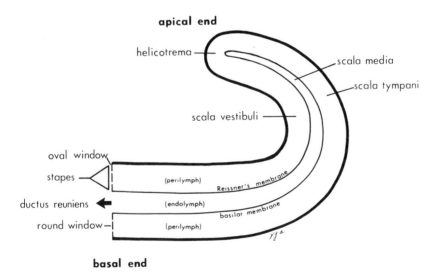

Figure 6.6.    An unrolled cochlea.

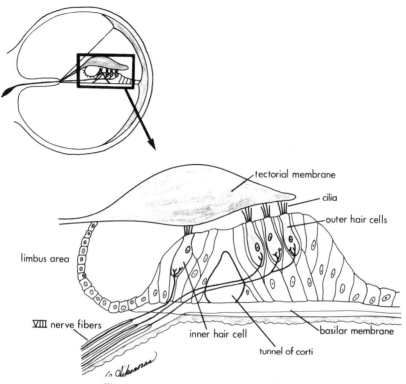

Figure 6.7.    Schematic of the organ of Corti.

very thin membrane, the *reticular lamina*. The reticular lamina has a series of perforations through which the cilia project. The tops of the cilia are embedded in the *tectorial membrane*, a jelly-like, colorless structure. The tectorial membrane is attached on its inner side to the upper lip of the bony spiral lamina in the region of the limbus.

We know that there are four rows of hair cells along the basilar membrane. There are about 3500 hair cells along the inner row and about 20,000 hair cells divided among the outer rows; the hair cells are fairly evenly spaced over the length of the membrane. The nerve fibers that innervate both the inner and outer hair cells group their cell bodies within the modiolus to form the *spiral ganglion of Corti*.

We should also note that the innervation patterns of both the inner and outer hair cells differ. Each inner hair cell is innervated by only one or two nerve fibers. Each outer hair cell is innervated by many fibers, and a single nerve fiber may innervate many hair cells.

The nerve fibers from the hair cells pass to the core of the modiolus, where they gather to form the *cochlear nerve,* one branch of the *VIII cranial* or *auditory nerve.* The fibers that form the cochlear nerve are not arranged haphazardly. Rather, they twist in conformity with the spirals of the cochlea. The end result is a core of fibers around which a rope-like pattern of fibers is wrapped. The core of the cochlear nerve contains those fibers that innervate the apical region of the cochlea. Those fibers that innervate the basal region of the cochlea are twisted about the core. Figure 6.4, a schematic diagram of a section through the cochlea, shows the arrangement of the nerve fibers in the modiolus and the separation of the VIII nerve.

The second portion of the VIII nerve, which is responsible for our sense of equilibrium, is known as the *vestibular nerve.* It arises from the *vestibular system,* which includes the three semicircular canals, and two membranous sacs in the vestibule known as the *utricle* and the *saccule.* The vestibular nerve joins the cochlear nerve just before the completed nerve enters the *internal auditory meatus,* a very narrow passage in the petrous portion of the temporal bone. As Figure 6.8 shows, the cochlear and vestibular nerves join just before the internal auditory meatus; also note how the VIII nerve branches to the various inner ear structures. The entire VIII cranial nerve is only about 4 mm to 5 mm (¼ inch) in length.

The VIII nerve terminates in the central nervous system. This occurs just after the nerve emerges from the internal auditory meatus. It enters

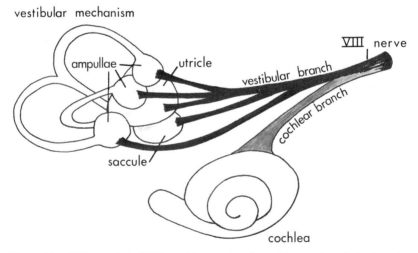

Figure 6.8.   Division of the VIII cranial nerve into its cochlear and vestibular branches.

the central nervous system in a region known as the *medulla*, a portion of the lower brainstem. The fibers then proceed to a mass of cell bodies in the brainstem known as the *cochlear nucleus*.

## THE VESTIBULAR SYSTEM

To review for a moment, we know that the bony labyrinth consists of the cochlea and the vestibular system. The former is responsible for our sense of hearing. The latter is responsible for our sense of balance or equilibrium. The vestibular system is similar to the cochlea in anatomy. It too is comprised of bony and membranous portions, the latter contained within the former. As was the case for the cochlea, the membranous portion of the vestibular system generally conforms to the overall shape of its bony counterpart; furthermore, there is no communication between the two systems. The spaces between the membranes and the bony walls are occupied by perilymph, and the spaces within the membranous portions are filled with endolymph. The actual sensory receptor cells are located within the membranous portion of the vestibular apparatus, just as they are in the membranous portion of the cochlea.

The vestibular apparatus consists of two main anatomical structures: the three semicircular canals, each of which is enlarged on one end, and the *otolith system*. This latter system consists of the utricle and the saccule. The membranous portion of the vestibular apparatus can be seen clearly in Figure 6.2.

The main purpose of the semicircular canals is to sense head motion or, more precisely, angular acceleration. For example, turning the head from side to side, or up and down, would cause sensory receptors (called *cristae*) located in the enlarged, or *ampullated*, ends of the semicircular canals to be stimulated. This action would then initiate a series of nerve impulses, which would ultimately arrive at the brain. The three semicircular canals are perpendicular to each other, making it possible to respond to all three directions in space.

The purpose of the otolith system is to sense linear acceleration. Such acceleration might be sensed when a car accelerates rapidly, or when one is moved upward or downward in an elevator. The sensory receptors in the utricle and saccule are called *maculae*.

## NEURONS AND NERVE CONDUCTION

In our discussion of the sensorineural mechanism we have mentioned such terms as *nerve fibers*, *cell bodies*, *ganglion cells*, and *receptors*. The fact that these terms were used presupposes some knowledge on the part of the reader of the structure of the nervous system. At this point, however, it may be worthwhile to briefly review the basics of nerve cells and nerve conduction.

The basic building block of the nervous system is the nerve cell, or *neuron*. A typical neuron is illustrated in Figure 6.9. As Figure 6.9 shows, a neuron has three distinct parts: the cell body or *soma*, the *dendrites*, and the *axon*. The function of the dendrites is to be stimulated by other neurons or by special receptors cells (such as the hair cells located in the cochlea or vestibular system). Thus, the dendrites act as the receiving ends of nerve cells, and they convey *nerve impulses* into the cell body. When discussing nervous system function, the term *affector* denotes reception of information. Thus, the dendrites act as affectors in nerve conduction.

Axons are long and thin extensions of the cell body. Their purpose is to act as *effectors*, or to convey information away from the cell bodies. The ends of the axons branch into much smaller fibers known as *terminal arbors* or end brushes. The terminal arbors, in turn, connect to other neurons across *synapses*. Thus, nerve impulses travel from neuron to neuron in a chain. In the case of the auditory system, there are at least four interconnecting neurons between the cochlea and the brain. The term *nerve fiber* may be applied to either dendrites or axons.

A group of cell bodies is referred to as a *nucleus* or a *ganglion*. If the cell bodies are outside the central nervous system (the brain and spinal cord), they generally take the name ganglion. Note, for example, the spiral ganglion of Corti. On the other hand, if the group of cell bodies

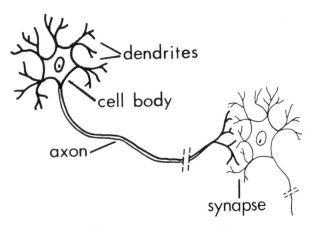

Figure 6.9.   Typical nerve cell.

lies within the central nervous system, the term *nucleus* is used. In the auditory system, the first grouping of cell bodies found in the central auditory nervous system is the cochlear nucleus.

What is a nerve impulse? The answer to this lies in the structure of the neuron itself. If we look at Figure 6.9, we see a thin membrane, the *myelin sheath*, surrounding the axon. The purpose of the sheath is to act as an electrical insulator between the axon, which maintains a small positive (+) electrical charge, and the surrounding chemical environment, which maintains a small negative (−) electrical charge. When the nerve fiber is in a state of rest, it acts like a miniature battery. That is, there is a minute voltage or potential which is maintained across the membrane. The membrane is said to be in a state of polarization. If the dendrites receive an incoming pulse of energy, and this pulse is of sufficient strength, the nerve fiber will "fire." When this occurs, a small portion of the membrane will depolarize, and that portion will momentarily conduct a minute flow of current. A wave of depolarization will then progress down the axon toward the terminal arbors. At the same time, those areas on the axon that were momentarily depolarized will, after a short rest or *refractory period*, become polarized once again. During the refractory period, the nerve is not capable of firing if stimulated.

## GLOSSARY

*afferent nerve*—A nerve that carries nerve impulses from a sensory organ to the central nervous system.

*axon*—Long extensions of nerve cells which carry information away from the cell body.

*basilar membrane*—Extends from the *osseous* (bony) spiral lamina to the outer wall of the cochlea, where it is held by the spiral ligament. The basilar membrane forms the upper side of the scala tympani, and also provides a base upon which the organ of Corti rests.

*bony labyrinth* (*osseous labyrinth*)—The actual hollowed-out form, within the temporal bone, of the series of communicating canals and cavities that comprise the labyrinth.

*bony spiral lamina*—A thin shelf of bone which partially divides the cochlea for most of its length.

*cochlear nerve*—The auditory branch of the VIII cranial or auditory nerve. The fibers that comprise the cochlear nerve arise from the spiral ganglion of Corti.

*cochlear nuclei*—Groups of cell bodies which receive the fibers from the cochlear nerve. They are located in the medulla.

*dendrites*—Small, finger-like processes of a nerve cell which carry nerve impulses to the cell body. They are the receiving ends of the neurons, or affectors.

*ductus reuniens*—A small membranous tube which unites the saccule with the scala media.

*efferent nerve*—A nerve that carries nervous impulses from the central nervous system to the periphery.

*endolymph*—The fluid that fills the membranous labyrinth.

*ganglion*—A collection of nerve cell bodies that have a common function but lie outside the central nervous system.

*hair cells*—Both the inner and outer hair cells are the actual receptor cells of acoustic stimuli within the cochlea. They derive their names from the hair-like structures, cilia, that project from their tops. There is a single row of inner hair cells and three rows of outer hair cells, which run down the basilar membrane.

*helicotrema*—A small opening, located at the apical end of the cochlea, that allows communication between the scala vestibuli and the scala tympani.

*internal auditory meatus*—A very small passage in the petrous portion of the temporal bone through which the VIII cranial (auditory) and VII cranial (facial) nerves pass on their way to the central nervous system.

*labyrinth*—The system of interconnecting canals and cavities within the temporal bone that makes up the inner ear. The labyrinth consists of the cochlea, the semicircular canals, and the vestibule.

*limbus*—A thickening of the fibrous membrane that covers the osseous spiral lamina.

*medulla*—The lowest part of the brainstem, extending from the pons to the spinal cord.

*membranous labyrinth*—A system of communicating membranous ducts and sacs which is contained within the larger bony labyrinth. The form of the membranous labyrinth generally conforms to the shape of the bony labyrinth. Contained within the membranous labyrinth are the sensory receptors for both the auditory and vestibular systems. Endolymph fills the membranous labyrinth.

*modiolus*—The central core of bone around which the cochlea turns for about 2¾ turns.

*myelin sheath*—A thin white sheath of fatty substance which surrounds the axons of most nerve fibers. Its purpose is to act as an insulator between the axon (which has a positive electrical charge) and the surrounding environment (which is negatively charged).

*nerve fiber*—Projections from the cell bodies of nerve cells. The term may be used for describing both dendrites and axons.

*nerve impulse*—A transient electrochemical change which rapidly sweeps from one end of a nerve fiber to the other. The impulse, once it reaches its termination at one fiber, may excite other fibers, muscles, or glands.

*neuron*—A nerve cell consists of a body (soma), an axon, and dendrites. Neurons are the basic units of the central nervous system.

*nucleus*—A collection of nerve cell bodies in the central nervous system that have a common feature.

*organ of Corti*—The actual sense organ of hearing, located on the upper surface of the basilar membrane, within the scala media.

*otolith system*—Consists of two membranous sacs, the utricle and the saccule, and is located within the vestibule. The otolith system is that part of the vestibular apparatus which responds to linear acceleration.

*oval window*—A small, oval-shaped opening which separates the middle from the inner ear. The window is closed by the stapes footplate and the annular ligament. The oval window terminates the scala vestibuli at its basal end.

*perilymph*—Perilymph is the fluid that fills the bony labyrinth.

*refractory period*—The refractory period of a nerve fiber is the time just after the fiber has been discharged. During this period, the fiber will not be fully charged and it will take a considerably stronger stimulus than usual to initiate a nerve impulse.

*Reissner's membrane*—The membrane that forms the base of the scala vestibuli and the upper side of the scala media. It extends diagonally from near the osseous spiral lamina to the outer cochlear wall.

*reticular lamina*—The reticular lamina is a thin membrane which lies on top of the hair cells in the organ of Corti. The ciliated ends of the hair cells perforate this membrane and then extend toward the tectorial membrane.

*round window*—A small round opening which separates the middle from the inner ear. Its membrane serves as the termination of the scala tympani at its basal end.

*saccule*—A membranous sac located within the vestibule. The saccule and utricle comprise the otolith system. The saccule communicates, through the ductus reuniens, with the scala media.

*scala media*—The scala media is triangular in cross section and is filled with endolymph. It is bounded by the scala vestibuli on its top side and by the scala tympani on its bottom side. The scala media is part of the membranous labyrinth and contains the organ of Corti. The scala media is also referred to as the *cochlear duct* or *cochlear partition*.

*scala tympani*—The lowermost channel in the cochlea. It is part of the bony labyrinth and contains perilymph. It is bounded on its upper side by the basilar membrane.

*scala vestibuli*—The uppermost channel in the cochlea. It is part of the bony labyrinth and is filled with perilymph. It is bounded on its lower side by Reissner's membrane.

*semicircular canals*—The portion of the inner ear that senses head motion. There are three canals, one for each dimension in space. The semicircular canals are part of the vestibular system.

*soma*—The cell body of a neuron.

*spiral ganglion of Corti*—The cell bodies of the neurons that innervate the hair cells of the cochlea. It is found in the modiolus and, as the name implies, this long ganglion spirals with the turns of the cochlea.

*spiral ligament*—A thick, fibrous membrane located on the outer wall of the cochlea, which holds the basilar membrane in place. The membrane is held on its other side by the osseous spiral lamina.

*stria vascularis*—A vascular layer of tissue which lines the outer wall of the scala media. The purpose of the stria vascularis is to secrete endolymph into the membranous labyrinth, as well as to be a blood supply to the cochlea.

*synapse*—The point at which a nerve impulse is passed from the axon of one nerve cell to the dendrites of another nerve cell; the junction of two neurons.

*tectorial membrane*—A jelly-like membrane which covers the organ of Corti. The cilia of the hair cells are embedded in the tectorial membrane.

*terminal arbors*—The branched ends of axons in a nerve cell.

*tunnel (canal) of Corti*—A supportive structure on the organ of Corti. It is formed by two pillars (the rods of Corti) which lean toward each other to form a triangle. This triangular structure, in turn, runs the entire length of the basilar membrane.

*utricle*—A membranous sac located within the vestibule. The utricle is part of the otolith system. It communicates with the semicircular canals.

*vestibular nerve*—The branch of the VIII cranial nerve responsible for the sense of equilibrium. The fibers arise from the otolith system and the semicircular canals.

*vestibule*—The central portion of the bony labyrinth which joins the cochlea to the semicircular canals. The otolith system, consisting of the *utricle* and *saccule*, is contained within the vestibule.

## SUGGESTED READING FOR FURTHER STUDY

Zemlin, W. R. 1968. *Speech and Hearing Science: Anatomy and Physiology.* Prentice-Hall, Englewood Cliffs, N.J.
A detailed account of the anatomy.

**STUDY QUESTIONS**

1. The central core of the cochlea is called the _____.
2. The three major portions of the bony labyrinth are the _____, _____, and _____.
3. The fluid in the membranous labyrinth is called _____.
4. The two major divisions of the VIII nerve are the _____ branch and the _____ branch.
5. The balance mechanism consists of the _____ and the _____.
6. The three channels of the cochlea are known as the _____, _____, and _____.
7. The actual sense organ of hearing, located in the cochlear duct, is the _____.
8. The sensory receptors that are located on the basilar membrane are known as _____.
9. The scala tympani terminates at the _____.
10. The labyrinth is a hollowed-out portion of the _____ bone.

# CHAPTER 7
# The Function and Dysfunction of the Sensorineural Mechanism

The primary function of the sensorineural mechanism is to conduct sound from the middle ear to the central nervous system, where it is integrated and interpreted. The sound collected at the footplate of the stapes is in the form of mechanical energy. The central nervous system only utilizes energy in the form of neurological impulses, which are electro-chemical in nature. Therefore, in order to deliver sound from the middle ear to the central nervous system, the sensorineural mechanism must *transduce* the energy from the mechanical energy into neurological impulses. This operation is performed within the cochlea, which, along with the VIII cranial nerve, comprises the sensorineural mechanism. The VIII nerve then transmits the neurological impulses to the brainstem, where they enter the auditory central nervous system.

## REVIEW OF COCHLEAR ANATOMY

The cochlea is a spiral-shaped organ that is divided into three fluid-filled tunnels or scalae within the temporal bone of the skull: *the scala vestibuli*, which begins in the vestibule near the oval window and winds through the basal, medial, and apical turns of the cochlea to the top of the cochlea, where it meets the scala tympani at the helicotrema and twists downward to the basal turn where it terminates at the round window membrane. These two passageways are separated by the scala media or cochlear partition; the cochlear partition is separated from the other scalae by Reissner's and the basilar membranes and contains the organ of Corti, which sits on the basilar membrane.

## PASSAGE OF SOUND VIBRATION
## FROM THE MIDDLE EAR TO THE VIII NERVE

### Fluid Displacement

The inward motion of the footplate of the stapes causes the displacement of a small amount of perilymph in the scala vestibuli. Since perilymph is nearly incompressible, the stapes movement causes a pressure wave to spread rapidly through the cochlea. In order to compensate for this pressure, the round window membrane is displaced outward into the middle ear cavity. During the outward movement phase of the stapes the elastic round window membrane returns to its resting position and the fluid flows back to its initial state.

Figure 7.1 is a simple schematic of an unrolled cochlea which will help us visualize the movement of fluid within the cochlea. From the diagram you can see that the simplest pattern of fluid displacement might be for the pressure wave caused by the footplate to travel up the scala vestibuli, through the very narrow helicotrema, and down the scala tympani to the round window. This pattern of fluid movement would leave the scala media unmoved. Since the organ of hearing is located within the scala media, such a fluid pattern would not provide for the transduction of mechanical energy into neurological impulses.

A more realistic and productive fluid pattern would have the pressure generated in the scala vestibuli transmitted across Reissner's membrane and the basilar membrane to the scala tympani, thereby distorting the entire cochlear partition (Figure 7.2). The pressure is released

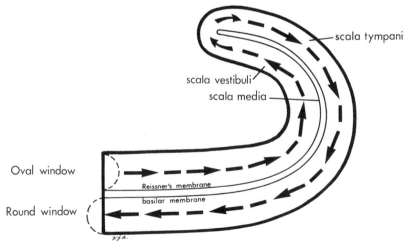

Figure 7.1.    Fluid displacement in the cochlea.

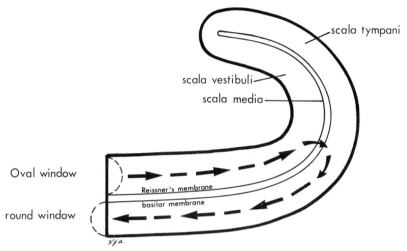

Figure 7.2.    Fluid displacement across the cochlear partition.

at the round window. Although the precise nature of fluid movement is still a matter of controversy, it is believed that the displacement of perilymph by the stapes causes a moving pressure wave in the cochlea. This is referred to as a *traveling wave*. The pressure bulge is transferred across the cochlear partition to the basilar membrane. The bulge moves or undulates along the basilar membrane from the basal turn toward the apical turn of the cochlea.

**Distortion of the Basilar Membrane**

The place in the cochlea where the maximum amplitude of the traveling wave occurs, thereby causing a point of maximal distortion of the basilar membrane, varies depending on the frequency of the input stimulus. Georg von Bekesy built a mechanical model of the cochlea and he was able to demonstrate that there was a direct relationship between the frequency of the stimulus and the anatomical location of the point of maximal displacement of the basilar membrane. He found that for high frequencies this point of maximal displacement occurs in the bottom of the cochlea, with the traveling wave dying out rapidly after the point of maximal displacement. Therefore, a high-frequency stimulus only stimulates the basal end of the cochlea. Lower frequencies spread throughout the cochlea, causing their maximal displacement toward the apex, thereby stimulating a much larger area of the cochlea. This geographical relationship with frequency in the cochlea is the basis of the *place theory of hearing*, which is discussed in more detail later in the chapter.

Figures 7.3 and 7.5 show the relationship between frequency and distance from the stapes in the cochlea. As you can see, the traveling

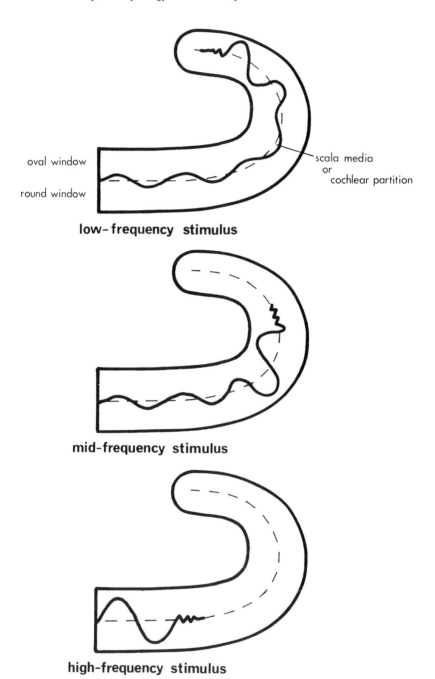

Figure 7.3.    Basilar membrane movement for high-, middle-, and low-frequency tones.

wave associated with a 2000-Hz stimulus causes its maximum distortion of the basilar membrane at approximately the midpoint of the cochlea before dissipating.

The relationship between frequency and displacement of the basilar membrane is determined by the anatomical structure of the membrane. The basilar membrane becomes notably wider as it progresses from the basal to the apical end of the cochlea, in spite of the fact that the cochlea itself becomes narrower. In addition, the membrane is also significantly less elastic at the basal end of the cochlea. These two factors cause the natural resonance of the basilar membrane to decrease as we move from the basal toward the apical turn. This accounts for the fact that different frequencies will cause the maximum point of displacement to occur at different points along the membrane.

In complex sounds, such as speech, the different component frequencies will cause multiple points of maximal displacement which correspond to the various component sine waves that combine to make the complex stimulus. In essence, the cochlea performs a filtering function, separating complex sounds into simple sine waves.

### Shearing Action of the Hair Cells

So far, we have said that the mechanical energy from the stapes is translated into a wave-like motion which crosses the cochlear partition and travels from the base of the cochlea upward along the basilar membrane. The organ of Corti is situated on the basilar membrane. The displacements of the membrane by the traveling wave are translated into up and down movments of the organ of Corti. It is important to remember that although both the basilar and tectorial membranes originate from the limbus area, they are hinged in distinctly different places (see Figure 6.5). The hair cells sit on the basilar membrane, but the ends of the cilia are attached to the tectorial membrane.

As the traveling wave passes along the basilar membrane, it causes a complex series of movements that involve not only up and down but also side to side and lengthwise displacements (Figure 7.4). Because the points of attachment are different for the basilar and tectorial membranes, the two structures do not move in concert, but actually slide in opposite directions. The end result is a complex twisting action of the hair cell cilia, which is referred to as the *shearing action.*

This mechanical shearing force, requiring the cilia to bend, causes the actual stimulation of the hair cells and the transduction of the mechanical energy into neurological impulses in the sensory nerve fibers, which are attached to the hair cells.

Bending the hair cells in only one direction will result in this stimulation; movements in the opposite direction will result in inhibition

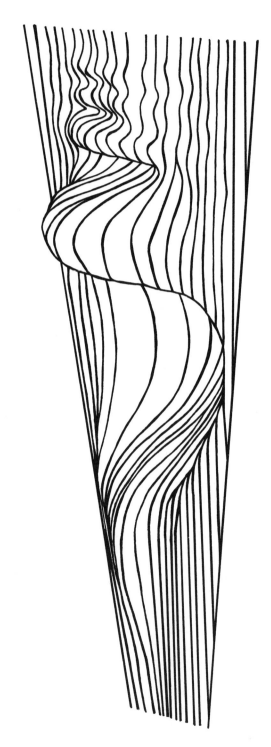

Figure 7.4. Traveling wave along the basilar membrane. (Adapted from Tonndorf, J. 1960. Dimensional analysis of cochlear models. *Journal of the Acoustical Society of America 32*: 493–497.)

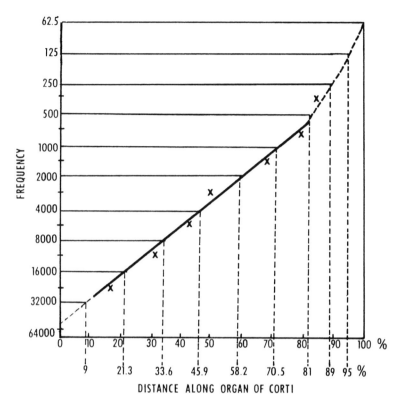

Figure 7.5.   Frequency map of the cochlea. (From Schuknecht, H. 1960. Neuroanatomical correlates of auditory sensitivity and pitch discrimination in the cat. In G. L. Rasmussen and W. F. Windle (eds.), *Neural Mechanisms of the Auditory and Vestibular Systems.* Charles C Thomas Publisher, Springfield, Ill.)

of nerve impulses. Sideways displacement of the cilia appears to have no effect.

## Cochlear Microphonic

One response of the organ of Corti to the shearing force is the generation of an alternating current (AC), known as the *cochlear microphonic*, which is believed to originate from the outer hair cells. The cochlear microphonic occurs only during the presence of acoustic stimulation of the ear, and is a faithful electrical mimic of the input sound until the stimulus reaches fairly high intensities (about 85 to 90 dB SPL). At high intensities the cochlear microphonic no longer corresponds on a one-to-one basis with the input stimulus, and actually degrades as the input intensity continues to increase. Although a great deal is not known about this, it appears to be related to overstimulation of the cochlea and may provide some insight into the temporary or permanent impairment of hair cell function that occurs following exposure to loud noise.

A new experimental technique called *electrocochleography* utilizes the cochlear microphonic to evaluate hearing in difficult-to-test patients.

## Hair Cell Transduction

The actual process responsible for the generation of neurological impulses in the sensory nerve fiber is still a matter of speculation. Some writers believe that the cochlear microphonic itself stimulates the nerve fibers to fire. Others believe that the cochlear microphonic is a by-product in the process, and that a chemical reaction at the base of the hair cell is essential to the transduction process. Still others believe that the simple mechanical distortion of the hair cells is responsible for generation of an impulse. In any case, the neurological impulse that is generated after a shearing action is carried by the auditory branch of the VIII cranial nerve to the central nervous system.

## THEORIES OF HEARING

The complex process that allows the ear to analyze and interpret the mechanical energy that the stapes delivers to the cochlea remains largely unknown. No simple theory has yet been advanced that accounts for all the facts, and most have focused primarily on pitch perception. Two distinct theories of hearing have been developed over the years: *place theory* and *frequency theory*.

Place theorists believe that the cochlea serves both as a transducer of energy and an analyzer of frequency and intensity. There can be little argument with the transducer role of the cochlea. Even though the pressure mechanism that allows the change of mechanical energy into neurological impulses may be subject to further definition, no serious student of audition doubts that transduction occurs in the organ of Corti at the time of the shearing action.

The second main tenet of place theory says that the cochlea is organized geographically according to frequency. In other words, for every frequency that the ear is able to perceive, there is a specific place in the cochlea that is sensitive to that frequency, as well as associated nerve fibers that carry the neurological message to the auditory central nervous system. This arrangement of the cochlea, VIII nerve, and auditory central nervous system is called *tonotopic organization*.

The contemporary form of place theory is Bekesy's *traveling wave theory*. Bekesy's experimental observations have indicated that a traveling wave is introduced to the cochlea by the movements of the stapes, and proceeds up the basilar membrane until it reaches a point of maximal amplitude. According to place theorists, only this point of maximal disturbance on the basilar membrane, whose location is determined by the frequency of the sound, is stimulated, and a neural message is sent through the VIII nerve to the auditory central nervous system. Therefore, the traveling wave theory, like all place theories, says that the cochlea acts as both an analyzer and transducer of sound.

Classical frequency theories argue that pitch and intensity analysis is a central process, and that the role of the cochlea is simply that of a transducer of mechanical energy into a neurological code that is entirely interpreted by the central nervous system; therefore frequency theorists hold that no tonotopic organization exists and the cochlea's only role is the transducer of energy.

Frequency theorists argue that pitch discrimination ability can be significantly improved with practice, proving that it is a learned behavior. Since learning is a central behavior and cannot be assigned to the peripheral organ, pitch discrimination cannot be a cochlear function. Early frequency theorists believed that the cochlea performed a simple coding operation that directly corresponded to the input signal: a 500-Hz stimulus yielded 500 nerve impulses per second. We now know, however, that an individual fiber in the auditory system is only capable of firing approximately 400 times per second. Since the human ear allows hearing of 20,000-Hz tones, this model is obviously unacceptable.

In attempting to modify classical frequency theory, Wever has suggested that a series of fibers could work in concert with each other to provide a continuous neurological message that would exceed the 400 impulse per second limit of the individual nerve fiber.

This cooperative firing of fibers is called the *volley principle* (Figure 7.6). Experimental evidence indicates that even with the use of the volley principle, only frequencies of up to 4000 Hz can be accounted for, leaving us far short of 20,000 Hz. Wever has suggested a combined place-frequency theory called the *volley theory* (it incorporates the volley principle), which suggests that both the spatial representation of the place theory and central interpretation of cochlear coding co-exist. The scope of this book does not allow an exhaustive discussion of hearing theory; the interested reader is referred to the supplementary readings at the conclusion of this chapter for further information.

## DISORDERS OF THE SENSORINEURAL MECHANISM

A hearing loss that occurs because of malfunctioning of the cochlea or VIII nerve is known as a sensorineural hearing loss. It is common

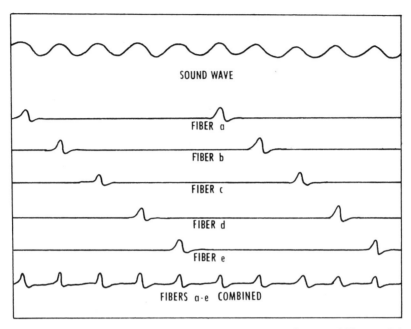

Figure 7.6   The volley principle. (From Wever, E. G. 1949. *Theories of Hearing.* John Wiley & Sons, Inc., New York.)

clinical practice to subdivide sensorineural disorders into *cochlear* and *retrocochlear* (along the pathway of the VIII nerve) hearing losses, depending on the location of the lesion causing the hearing loss.

If a hearing loss is caused by damage to the auditory mechanism that occurs before birth, the loss is referred to as *congenital*, as opposed to *acquired hearing losses*, which develop any time postnatally.

## Congenital Hearing Loss

One of the most common forms of deafness is genetically transmitted hearing loss. These hereditary losses can occur as part of a pattern of symptoms called a *syndrome*, or in isolation, where the hearing loss is the only abnormality present.

Such genetically transmitted hearing losses may be dominant or recessive, and the hearing loss that results may vary from mild to profound.

Although in most cases the hearing loss associated with hereditary disorders is present at birth, we now recognize the existence of genetically transmitted degenerative hearing losses, where hearing abnormalities are predetermined to occur later in life. Even if one were able to know of an impending postnatal hereditary hearing loss, prevention would be impossible, and the audiologist must rely on early identification and appropriate therapy.

A variety of nonhereditary problems can occur during the prenatal period that may affect the normal development of hearing.

Until recently Rh incompatibility was a major causative factor in prenatal hearing loss. The problem occurs only when an Rh+ fetus is produced from the union of an Rh− mother and an Rh+ father. Rh+ means that a protein molecule called Rh is present in the blood supply. The mother produces antibodies to protect herself against the Rh factor, which is foreign to her system; the concentration, and therefore the potential damage to the fetus from these antibodies, increases with each successive pregnancy. The incidence of Rh-related disorders has decreased greatly in recent years as physicians have developed methods of preventing the maternal development of Rh antibodies following pregnancy, and of transfusing infants' blood to remove Rh antibodies before the damage can occur.

*Rubella* (German measles) is of minimal concern to an adult afflicted with it; but this virus infection is a matter of great concern when contracted by a pregnant woman. Although the danger is greatest during the first 3 months of pregnancy, injury to the fetus can also occur much later in pregnancy. The most common effects of maternal rubella are brain damage, heart defects, visual defects, and sensorineural hearing loss, occurring individually or, often, in combination.

A vaccine has been developed to prevent rubella; successful control of this disease, as with polio, remains a public health administrative problem.

Drugs that are ingested by a pregnant woman may affect the hearing of the fetus, although research in this area is often inconclusive. For example, the damaging effects of quinine and thalidomide are well known, although the effects of the use of a variety of commonly used illegal drugs are not well researched.

*Anoxia*, the lack of sufficient oxygen during the birth process, is a common cause of central nervous system damage and sometimes may result in sensorineural hearing loss. Anoxia is often associated with premature delivery, head trauma to the baby during delivery, or an umbilical cord twisted around the neck of the fetus.

## Acquired Sensorineural Hearing Loss

**Infections**   Both viral and bacterial infections can result in damage to the sensorineural mechanism. These hearing losses can be unilateral or bilateral, and can vary in degree from mild to total loss of hearing.

A bacterial or viral infection of the inner ear is called *labyrinthitis*, and is usually associated with vertigo as well as hearing loss, since the vestibular mechanism is also involved.

An infection of the brain covering is known as *meningitis*. Should the infection travel to the inner ear, it can do widespread damage to the cochlea and VIII nerve.

Although many of the common childhood diseases have been linked to sensorineural damage, only mumps and measles are frequently associated with hearing loss. Although most viral-related hearing losses are bilateral, some, for example the mumps, are associated with unilateral losses.

The high fevers that occur with infections are sometimes blamed for cochlear damage, although the cause of the fever cannot be eliminated as a possible etiology. Sometimes, otherwise asymptomatic viruses can cause sudden unilateral or bilateral hearing losses in children and adults, although the specific etiology is often unknown.

Sudden onset hearing losses can also be precipitated by interruptions of the blood supply to the cochlea. As in sudden viral attacks, the symptoms may disappear spontaneously, but often the sensorineural hearing loss is not reversible.

Sensorineural hearing loss is one of the many severe consequences of *syphilis*; others are brain damage, blindness, and sometimes death. In addition to acquired syphilis, which consistently appears to evade public health control efforts, congenital syphilis must be considered a significant prenatal factor in hearing loss.

**Ototoxic Drugs**   Some drugs are associated with sensorineural damage to the ear. The most important of these are kanamycin, dihydrostreptomycin, neomycin, vancomycin, gentamycin, and streptomycin, which should be used by the physician in extreme circumstances when other drug choices are not feasible.

Aspirin, in prolonged use, is also known to be ototoxic, but its effects are often at least partially reversible when the drug is withdrawn. Quinine, which is used to treat malaria, is also known to cause sensorineural hearing loss. Patients who have impaired renal (kidney) function are particularly susceptible to all ototoxicity, because the drug is allowed to remain in the patient's system long after it should have been excreted by a normal kidney function.

**Ménière's Disease**   The symptoms of Ménière's disease are tinnitus, progressive sensorineural hearing loss, which is usually unilateral, and sudden attacks of vertigo and nausea. Many researchers believe that Ménière's disease is due to the presence of excessive endolymph in the membranous labyrinth. The excess pressure in the cochlea causes tinnitus and hearing loss; this pressure also affects the vestibular mechanism, causing the vertigo.

Ménière's disease may become very extreme and actually may make normal living impossible. Some patients find they are unable to work or drive a car. In such extreme cases it may be necessary to sever the auditory nerve or destroy the affected labyrinth, despite the total loss of hearing on that side, in order to eliminate the debilitating effects of the disease.

**Trauma**    Although the tympanic membrane and the ossicular chain are far more susceptible to damage from blows to the head, contusions to the cochlea and skull fracture through the cochlear area may result in sensorineural hearing loss.

**VIII Nerve Tumors**    Space-occupying lesions can develop along the course of the VIII nerve from the cochlea to the brainstem. These slow-growing tumors are almost always benign and are very dangerous because as they grow, they cause increased intracranial pressure. They are most commonly found in the internal auditory meatus (IAM) or at the cerebellopontine angle. Surgical removal is the only treatment available.

**Noise-Induced Hearing Loss**    It has long been recognized that exposure to loud noise can be detrimental to one's hearing levels. In addition to auditory effects, intense noise has been demonstrated to lead to a variety of adverse psychological and physiological effects, such as anxiety and loss of attention span.

Exposure to noises in excess of 85 dB SPL must be considered dangerous, although individual susceptibility to acoustic trauma varies greatly from person to person.

A sudden acoustic trauma, such as an explosion, may result in permanent sensorineural hearing loss. Often this loss will primarily affect the 3000- to 6000-Hz frequency range, although more severe damage may result in a hearing loss at all frequencies.

Noise-induced hearing loss may progress slowly, such as in work-related noise exposure. Initial exposure to noise usually results in a loss of hearing in the 3000- to 6000-Hz range, which disappears a number of hours after the noise exposure ends. This is referred to as a *temporary threshold shift* (TTS). Gradually, with continued exposure, the loss also begins to affect the lower frequencies as well and hearing does not return to normal after a rest period from the noise exposure; this is now referred to as a *permanent threshold shift* (PTS).

The patient who shows the initial effects of a noise-induced hearing loss must protect his or her hearing with the use of earplugs or earmuffs. Counseling is extremely important because the effects are often gradual and the patient is frequently unaware of the severity of the problem.

**Presbycusis**    The loss of hearing associated with the aging process is called *presbycusis*. The hearing loss that accompanies it is both sensorineural and central in nature. Presbycusis usually involves a progressive sensorineural hearing loss that tends to be worse in the higher frequencies, and a loss of auditory discrimination ability that is often more troublesome to the patient than the loss of sensitivity. Furthermore, the many behavioral changes associated with aging often complicate the problem and make the rehabilitation of the geriatric patient a difficult and challenging process for the audiologist.


## GLOSSARY

*acquired hearing loss*—One that is acquired, for various reasons, after birth. Noise exposure, disease, head trauma, presbycusis, and ototoxic drugs are possible causes.

*anoxia*—The absence of oxygen.

*cochlear hearing loss*—One in which the site of the hearing disorder is within the cochlea itself.

*cochlear microphonic*—An electrical potential which may be recorded from various places in the cochlea. The microphonic closely resembles the waveforms of the sounds that enter the ears. It is thought that the cochlear microphonic originates in the hairs of the hair cells, and serves to stimulate the auditory nerve fibers which innervate the hair cells.

*congenital hearing loss*—One that existed before birth. Congenital hearing loss may be either hereditary or acquired in utero.

*electrocochleography* (*ECoG*)—A clinical electrophysiological procedure that records electrical responses of the cochlea and auditory nerve to various acoustic signals.

*frequency theory of hearing*—Theory of hearing in which the analysis of pitch is thought to occur at the cerebral level; the cochlea simply acts to transduce the acoustic signals to an appropriate neural code which the brain interprets.

*labyrinthitis*—A general term which refers to an inflammation of the inner ear. The condition is associated with vertigo and hearing loss.

*meningitis*—An inflammation of the membranes that cover the brain, or of the spinal cord.

*permanent threshold shift* (*PTS*)—Refers to a permanent reduction of auditory sensitivity after exposure to intense sound.

*place theory of hearing*—A theory of hearing in which the analysis of pitch is thought to occur in the cochlea; the brain acts as a receiver of the already decoded auditory messages.

*retrocochlear hearing loss*—A hearing loss in which the auditory dysfunction is located along the path of the auditory nerve (VIII cranial nerve).

*rubella*—Also popularly known as "German measles." It is an acute viral disease, usually mild in degree. It most often occurs in children and young adults, and is characterized by a pale pink rash. If a pregnant woman contracts rubella, primarily in the first trimester of pregnancy, the fetus may develop a number of congenital defects. These include hearing loss, cardiovascular defects, and visual difficulties.

*shearing action*—Refers to the mechanical bending of the hair cells on the organ of Corti by the tectorial membrane as the fluids in the cochlea move.

*syndrome*—A set of symptoms that characterize a disease.

*syphilis*—An infectious and chronic venereal disease which is transmitted either by direct contact or congenitally.

*temporary threshold shift (TTS)*—A temporary reduction in hearing sensitivity following exposure to intense noise.

*tonotopic organization*—The orderly arrangement of auditory centers in the auditory central nervous system, such that each center would be arranged as a frequency map of the cochlea. Thus, the frequency arrangement of the cochlea would, if tonotopically organized, be unrolled at other levels in the auditory system.

*transducer*—A device that changes energy from one form to another, thus allowing energy to flow from one system to another.

*traveling wave*—The wave of basilar membrane motion from base to apex. The site of maximum stimulation of the basilar membrane changes with frequency. It is close to the base for high frequencies, and moves progressively toward the apex for lower frequencies.

## SUGGESTED READINGS FOR FURTHER STUDY

Harris, J. D. 1974. *Anatomy and Physiology of the Peripheral Hearing Mechanism*, pp. 39–52. Bobbs-Merrill Company, Inc., Indianapolis.
A brief account of cochlear function.
Littler, T. S. 1965. *The Physics of the Ear*, Chapter 4. Pergamon Press, Oxford.
A detailed account of cochlear function.
von Bekesy, G. 1960. *Experiments in Hearing*. McGraw-Hill Book Company, New York.
A classic work in the field of hearing by a Nobel Prize winner.
Wever, E. G., and M. Lawrence. 1954. *Physiological Acoustics*. Princeton University Press, Princeton.
Complete and readable account of theories of hearing.

## STUDY QUESTIONS

1. The cochlea and the auditory nerve comprise the _____ mechanism.
2. The transduction of the auditory stimulus into neurological impulses takes place in the _____.
3. Movement of the stapes stimulates the basilar membrane in the form of a _____.
4. High-frequency sounds cause the stimulation of hair cells in the _____ turn of the cochlea.
5. A _____ theory of hearing states that the cochlea functions both as a transducer and analyzer of sound.
6. An electrical response from the hair cells, which mimics the input auditory stimulus, is called the _____.
7. Hearing loss associated with aging is called _____.
8. A lesion along the VIII nerve may produce a _____ type of hearing loss.
9. A viral disease that may cause hearing loss in the fetus if contracted in the first trimester of pregnancy is _____.
10. A disorder characterized by unilateral sensorineural loss and episodes of vertigo is _____.

# CHAPTER 8
# The Central Auditory Mechanism

We have studied the role of the conductive and sensorineural mechanisms in the hearing process. The sound energy has been transduced by the cochlea into neurological impulses which are carried from the cochlea to the beginning of the central auditory nervous system in the brainstem by the auditory portion of the VIII nerve.

En route from the cochlea, the auditory portion of the VIII nerve joins the vestibular portion of the VIII nerve and passes through the internal auditory meatus. The VII or facial nerve also passes through the internal auditory meatus on the way to the brainstem. The auditory nerve extends a very short distance beyond the internal auditory meatus before joining the brainstem at an angle formed by the cerebellum and the pons (the *cerebellopontine angle*). The fibers of the auditory branch then run to a way station called the *cochlear nucleus*, which marks the beginning of the auditory central nervous system.

In the central nervous system the anatomy and physiology are very intricate and complex and our understanding is far from complete. We will present a simplified outline of the neuroanatomy, tracing the pathway of a neurological impulse from the VIII nerve to the auditory cortex and labeling each of the neurological way stations or *synapses* we encounter as we ascend from the cochlea to the auditory cortex.

Such an ascending pathway for neurological impulses is referred to as an *afferent pathway* or tract, in opposition to a descending pathway from the cortex toward the periphery, which is called an *efferent pathway*.

## REVIEW OF THE GROSS ANATOMY

The brainstem (Figure 8.1) consists primarily of the medulla, which is continuous with the spinal cord on its underside; the pons, which is above the medulla; and the midbrain, which is above the pons.

The cortex is made up of two cerebral hemispheres which are partially separated by a deep fissure and interconnected by a system of

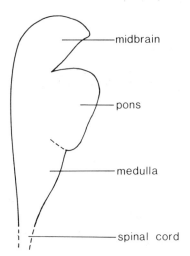

Figure 8.1.    Schematic of the brainstem.

nerve fibers. Each of the hemispheres is divided into four areas, called lobes (Figure 8.2).

The *thalamus* lies in a portion of the brain called the *diencephalon*. The diencephalon is like the core of the brain. It is above the midbrain and completely surrounded by the cerebral hemispheres.

### THE AFFERENT CENTRAL AUDITORY PATHWAY

Let us first consider just one ear, as is shown in Figure 8.3. The afferent neurological fibers of the VIII nerve terminate at the cochlear nucleus, which is in the medulla. From this way station, two ascending pathways or tracts can be seen. The pathway on the same side of the brainstem as the cochlea in Figure 8.3 is called the *ipsilateral* pathway, and the pathway on the other side of the brainstem is called the *contralateral* pathway. Approximately two-thirds of the fibers from the cochlear nucleus cross over the brainstem (decussate) on the way to the next way station, the *superior olivary complex*, which is also in the medulla. The remaining one-third of the fibers ascend to the superior olivary complex on the ipsilateral side. In addition to being a neural way station, the superior olivary complex controls the activity of both middle ear muscle reflexes. When the neurological impulses from loud sounds arrive at the superior olivary complex (via the VIII nerve), messages are sent down the VIII nerve to the stapedius muscle and down the V (trigeminal) nerve to the tensor tympani muscle causing contraction of thése muscles in the middle ear.

Moving upward in Figure 8.3, the next way station in the central auditory tract is the nucleus of the lateral lemniscus in the pons. From there, the next way station is the inferior colliculus in the midbrain.

The two inferior colliculi are connected by fibers that allow crossover from one side of the brainstem to the other.

Some fibers from the lateral lemniscus bypass the inferior colliculi and ascend directly to the next way station, the *medial geniculate body*, which is located in the thalamus. After this point, the tract fans out into multiple small fibers known as the *auditory radiations*, which connect the medial geniculate body to the auditory cortex in the temporal lobe.

The auditory reception areas are located in both temporal lobes. Although such high-level behaviors as the understanding of speech and processing other complex signals require the integrity of the auditory cortex, perception of loudness and pitch and many other simpler auditory behaviors are dealt with on the brainstem level.

**TWO-EAR REPRESENTATION**

Figure 8.3 only shows the pathway for a single ear. Figure 8.4 is essentially the same diagram, with input indicated from both ears. From the superior olivary complex upward, both the ipsilateral and con-

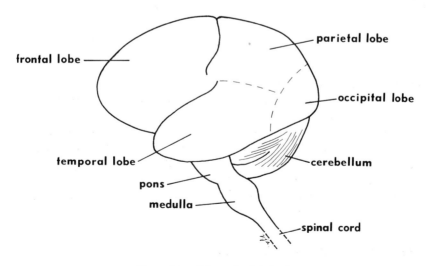

Figure 8.2.   Schematic of the brain.

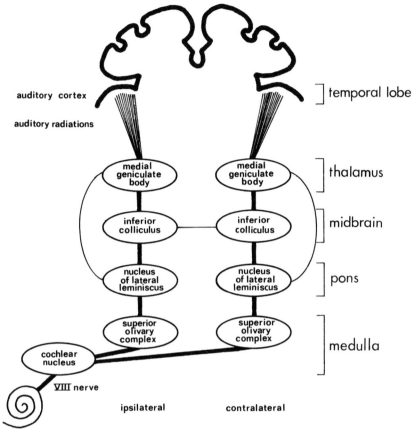

Figure 8.3.   Central auditory pathway for the left ear. (Illustration by Valerie Aiksnoras.)

tralateral tracts contain information from both ears. It is important to understand that what is contralateral for the right ear is ipsilateral for the left ear and vice versa.

The first point at which hearing from both ears is represented in the central auditory system is the superior olivary complex. We know that, in addition to the earlier mentioned functions of this way station, the superior olivary complex is responsible for the ability to localize sounds in space, a behavior that requires comparison of the information received from both ears (see Chapter 10).

### EFFERENT AUDITORY PATHWAY

Although the auditory pathway is primarily thought of as an ascending sensory pathway, there is also known to be an efferent pathway of descending fibers that originates in the temporal lobe and goes all the way back through the brainstem to the organ of Corti. An important part of this efferent system is known as the *olivo-cochlear bundle*, which descends from the superior olivary complex to the organ of Corti.

The efferent auditory system is not well understood but is known to provide an inhibitory function that can result in a significant increase in the intensity needed to hear a stimulus. This may be related to our ability to "tune out" the auditory input under certain conditions.

## SUMMARY

The major pathways from the cochlea to the auditory cortex have been described. Much is not known about the specific functions that are car-

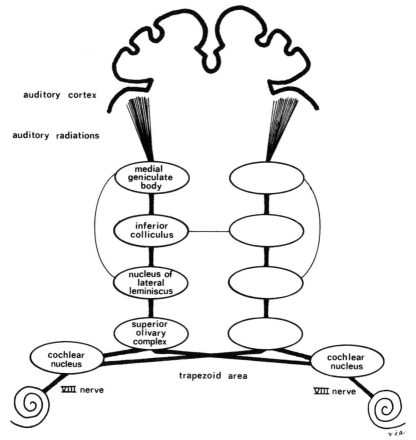

Figure 8.4.    Schematic of the central auditory pathway. (Illustration by Valerie Aiksnoras.)

ried on at each way station, and still less is understood about the actual processing and utilization of the auditory input in the cortex.

## DISORDERS OF THE CENTRAL AUDITORY SYSTEM

Although a lengthy discussion of the disorders of the central auditory system is beyond the scope of this book, it is important to distinguish a *central hearing loss* from a *peripheral* (conductive or sensorineural) *hearing loss*. A central hearing loss manifests itself as a problem in interpretation, integration, and/or appropriate utilization of the auditory input. Unlike a peripheral disorder, the patient will not normally have the loss of hearing sensitivity that we usually associate with hearing disorders. For this reason, a central hearing loss is probably more appropriately referred to as central dysacusis.

The symptoms of a central hearing disorder are often vague and difficult to define. The correlation of the symptoms with specific anatomical damage is often impossible. Sometimes the damage is a clearly localized lesion, like a tumor in the brain or brainstem; at other times the damage is diffuse, as in *arteriosclerosis*. The patient's symptoms can vary from difficult-to-define auditory perceptual problems to severe *auditory agnosia*, a loss of the ability to recognize familiar auditory stimuli.

In increasing numbers, audiologists are becoming involved in central auditory evaluation. The standard audiological methods rarely provide meaningful information because they are directed at identifying losses of hearing sensitivity. Complex speech stimuli, such as speeded speech and frequency-distorted speech, and tests that involve the use of competing message material have proved useful in identifying disorders of the central auditory system. Certainly, the identification and differentiation of auditory disorders of the brain and brainstem is one of the most rapidly developing areas in audiology at present.

## GLOSSARY

*afferent pathway*—Conducts nerve impulses toward the brain. Another term for afferent pathway is *ascending tract*.

*arteriosclerosis*—A condition in which degenerative changes in the arteries cause a thickening and hardening of the arterial walls, decreasing the blood supply.

*auditory agnosia*—The inability to recognize auditory stimuli, even though sensitivity may fall within normal limits.

*auditory radiations*—A large bundle of small fibers which runs from the medial geniculate body to the auditory cortex.

*central hearing loss*—Caused by a lesion that involves either the auditory pathways from the brainstem to the medial geniculate body, or the auditory centers of the cortex, or both.

*decussate*—A nerve that decussates crosses over from one side of the brainstem or brain to the other.

*efferent pathway*—Conducts nerve impulses away from the brain to the periphery. Another term for efferent pathway is *descending tract*.

*medial geniculate body*—The last auditory relay station before the auditory cortex. The medial geniculate body is located on the *thalamus*. It receives its auditory impulses through the inferior colliculus, and then sends the impulses to the cortex by way of the *auditory radiations*.

*thalamus*—An intricate relay station through which nerve impulses pass on their way to and from the cortex.

## SUGGESTED READINGS FOR FURTHER STUDY

Davis, H., and S. R. Silverman. 1978. *Hearing and Deafness*, Chapter 3. 4th Ed. Holt, Rinehart & Winston, Inc., New York.
A well-written introduction.
Martin, F. N. 1975. *Introduction to Audiology*, Chapter 9. Prentice-Hall, Englewood Cliffs, N.J.
A good overview for the beginning audiologist.
Yost, W. A., and D. W. Nielsen. 1977. *Fundamentals of Hearing: An Introduction*, Chapter 7. Holt, Rinehart & Winston, Inc., New York.
A more complete treatment.

## STUDY QUESTIONS

1. The junction between two nerve fibers is called a _____.
2. The lowest portion of the brainstem is called the _____.
3. An ascending tract that carries information from the periphery to the cortex is called an _____ pathway.
4. The crossover of nerve fibers from one side to the other is called _____.
5. The central auditory pathway terminates in the _____ lobe of the brain.
6. The junction formed by the cerebellum and the pons is called the _____ angle.
7. The middle ear muscle reflexes are mediated in the central nervous system at the _____.
8. The loss of the ability to recognize familiar sounds is known as _____.
9. The location where the sensorineural and central systems join is the _____.
10. The small, finger-like nerve fibers which terminate at the auditory cortex are called _____.

# PART III
## THE PERCEPTION
## OF SOUND

# CHAPTER 9
# Normal Hearing

The most fundamental question one can ask in the science of hearing is: "What is the softest sound that can be heard?" Although the human ear is amazingly sensitive to a wide variety of acoustic stimuli, we all know that sounds exist that we cannot hear, such as a high-frequency dog whistle. There are many reasons why some sounds are not audible. For example, the sound may be too weak in intensity, or the sound may lie outside the frequency range that the ear is sensitive to. The sound may be overshadowed (masked) by competing environmental noise. Finally, the sound may not be attended to by the listener, and therefore is unheard. Some people are not able to hear sounds that are audible to most others and are said to have a hearing loss.

The basic measure in audition is the threshold, or the minimum intensity at which a stimulus is barely audible. The threshold level is determined by both the sensitivity of the auditory mechanism and the nature of the stimulus used to elicit a response.

This chapter focuses on two main topics that are essential to the clinician if he is to use the threshold concept meaningfully:

1. The variables affecting the minimal auditory stimulus. These include acoustic parameters of the signal, methodological variables, and psychological factors affecting the listener.
2. The concept of normal hearing and hearing loss and the measurement and differentiation of types of hearing loss.

## ACOUSTIC FACTORS

### Frequency

The human ear is responsive to a wide range of frequencies, varying from about 20 Hz to 20,000 Hz. However, it is not equally sensitive across this range; in order to hear some frequencies one must provide a stimulus of great intensity and at other frequencies we can perceive rather small intensities. Human hearing is most sensitive in the 1000- to 3000-Hz range. Hearing sensitivity for the lower frequencies drops off notably as frequency decreases below 500 Hz toward the lower limits of hearing. A similar but less dramatic effect can be seen from about 3000 to 12,000 Hz; hearing sensitivity then drops sharply until we reach the upper limits of audition.

Figure 9.1 is a graphic representation of the average sensitivity of the human ear from 125 to 8000 Hz for a normal group of hearers. In the normal ear the threshold for a 1000-Hz tone is 7 dB SPL. However, at 125 Hz, the same normal listener requires 45 dB SPL, a far greater intensity, to first perceive the tone. At 8000 Hz, one needs 13 dB SPL to reach threshold.

**Lower Frequency Limit**     The lower frequency limit of hearing is difficult to define because very low frequency stimuli cause both auditory and tactile stimulation, which are often difficult to separate. This is apparent when we listen to loud music and "feel" our skin tingle in response to some loud bass notes. In addition, it is acoustically difficult to provide intense stimuli at low frequencies that are free of harmonics. Since hearing is far more acute at 60 Hz, for example, than at 30 Hz, a 30-Hz stimulus with harmonic energy that is audible at 60 Hz may provide very misleading data. Depending on the method employed and the definition of hearing that is accepted, most research indicates that the lower limit of audition lies somewhere between 10 and 30 Hz.

**Upper Frequency Limit**     There has been much research on the upper limit of hearing; the main confounding variable in this area is the appropriate generation of the stimulus. Hearing has been demonstrated in young normal subjects up to 23,000 Hz. At these frequencies a great

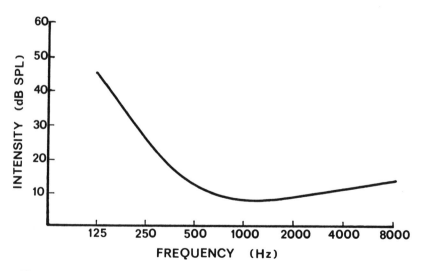

Figure 9.1.   Normal human hearing (American National Standards Institute—ANSI).

deal of intensity is needed for the tone to be heard; for example, an 18,000-Hz tone requires about 70 dB SPL of intensity to reach threshold in young subjects.

**Time Factors**

If the tone used is about 200 milliseconds ($\frac{1}{5}$ second) or longer, duration is not a significant factor in determining the minimal audible stimulus. However, as the stimulus duration is reduced below 200 milliseconds, the intensity needed for the ear to just perceive a pure tone is increased significantly. The shorter the stimulus duration, the greater intensity that will be needed to reach threshold. Figure 9.2 illustrates the relationship between stimulus duration and threshold for pure tones. Between 5 and 13 dB of additional intensity are needed as the tone duration is reduced from 500 to 16 milliseconds. Note that this temporal effect is more pronounced in the lower frequencies.

The effect of stimulus duration on threshold level is usually referred to as *temporal integration*, or summation. The auditory system appears to be able to summate and integrate energy over a maximal period of about 200 to 250 milliseconds. What occurs is that the auditory system is able to maintain a threshold level as long as increased intensity makes up for decreases in duration. This trade between time and intensity, however, only occurs at durations of about 200 milliseconds and less. Figure 9.2 shows that if the duration is increased above 200 to 250 milliseconds, the threshold level remains constant. In other words, the tone duration is not related to threshold level, or there is no temporal summation. In audiology, tones of approximately one-half (500 milliseconds) to a full second (1000 milliseconds) are used as stimuli to reduce the effects of tone durations on thresholds.

**Method of Measurement**

In defining the threshold for a given tone, the procedure used in obtaining the measurement is an important variable. Two methods of presenting stimuli are commonly used in determining auditory threshold measurements: minimal audible field (MAF) and minimal audible pressure (MAP).

**Minimal Audible Field**   In some experiments the stimuli are presented in a special room with a controlled sound environment called a sound field. All stimulus parameters are determined in a position that corresponds to the position of the listener's head when he or she is not in the sound field. Threshold values are then collected with the subject positioned in the sound field environment; these measurements are referred to as *minimum audible field* (*MAF*) data. The MAF technique is

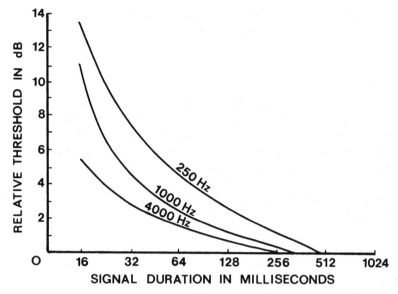

Figure 9.2.   Thresholds as a function of stimulus duration.

reasonably analogous to a normal listening situation, but a number of variables that are inherent in the method must be considered. The position of the head in the sound field affects sound reflections in the area of the two ears; this is known as the *head shadow effect*. The size of this effect is determined by the angle of the head to the sound source and the frequency of the stimulus used; this is discussed more fully in Chapter 10 on binaural hearing. The placing of the subject's body in the sound field also affects the measurements; these perturbations on the stimulus are referred to as the *body baffle effect*. The ear canal also has a *resonance effect*, which modifies the signal from the source before it reaches the tympanic membrane. The external auditory meatus has a natural resonance in the area of 3500 Hz; this resonance can amplify sound in the range of 3000 to 4500 Hz as much as 10 dB. The literature shows the sum of all these effects in the sound field (body baffle, head shadow, and canal resonance) can cause amplification of a stimulus in the 3000- to 8000-Hz range of up to 20 dB. This is especially significant because this is the critical area for the understanding of speech sounds.

**Minimal Audible Pressure**   Measurements that are obtained by delivering the stimuli through earphones are known as *minimal audible pressure (MAP)* measures. Although this situation may not have the apparent correlation to everyday listening situations that MAF does, the earphone technique has many advantages for research and clinical purposes. It is far easier to build an adequate sound-treated room to allow earphone (MAP) measurements than it is to build a properly controlled anechoic (echo-free) sound field for MAF measurements.

It is relatively simple to obtain accurate acoustic measurements in an earphone situation. Calibration measurement is accomplished using a standardized mechanical device known as a *coupler*, which approximates the air volume (6 cc) trapped between the earphone cushion and the tympanic membrane. The intensity of the stimulus is measured by a sound level meter (SLM), which is attached to the earphone through the coupler; this arrangement is often referred to as an artificial ear (Figure 9.3). For experimental purposes, it is also possible to slip a probe-tube microphone under the earphone cushion to the region of the tympanic membrane in order to obtain acoustic calibration data. This technique is almost never used in the clinic but is more often reserved for highly accurate research studies.

Figure 9.4 shows a comparison of hearing thresholds obtained by MAF and MAP methods. It can be seen that hearing is about 5 to 7 dB better when measured by MAF technique. Note that the general frequency contour is essentially unchanged, with most sensitive hearing lying between 1000 and 3000 Hz.

**Psychophysical Methods**

Aside from the technique used to present the stimuli, the method of threshold measurement is an important variable in the data obtained. There are three principal psychophysical methods used to determine threshold; the *method of limits*, the *method of adjustment*, and the *method of constant stimuli*. The last is quite time consuming and not normally applied to clinical measures of threshold. In the method of limits, the tester gradually increases or decreases the intensity of the stimulus from audibility to inaudibility (or vice versa) and records the subject's responses. In the method of adjustment, the subject controls the stimulus intensity and sets it according to the tester's directions, such as "barely audible." A modified method of limits procedure is adopted for pure tone threshold determination in audiology, while the Bekesy test technique utilizes the method of adjustment.

Threshold data will be affected if the stimuli are presented ascending from inaudibility to audibility or descending from audibility to inaudibility. For tones, a descending series tends to produce a higher threshold than an ascending series.

**AGE**

Hearing sensitivity is known to decrease with advancing age, with the higher frequencies generally being affected first and more severely.

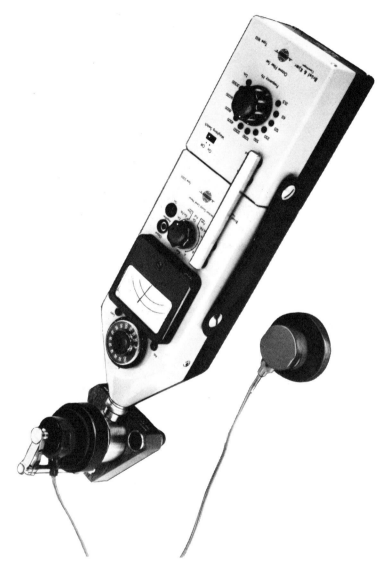

Figure 9.3.　Artificial ear. (Courtesy of Bruel & Kjaer, Inc.)

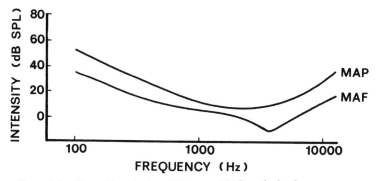

Figure 9.4.   Normal hearing by MAF versus MAP methods of measurement.

Studies show that hearing is most sensitive at about age 12 and slowly decreases as part of the  physiological process of aging. This hearing loss with aging is known as *presbycusis*; the degree of impairment varies widely from individual to individual, with some persons showing little effect of aging on their thresholds. Women show less high-frequency hearing loss as a function of age than men. Many researchers believe that there is a causal relationship between presbycusis and long-term noise exposure. Women generally are exposed to lower occupational noise levels than men, providing a logical, but unproven, hypothesis to account for the difference.

Figure 9.5 illustrates the effect of age on hearing level as a function of frequency. As you can see, the effect is most striking at 6000 Hz, where hearing decreases from a mean of approximately 10 dB at age 40 to about

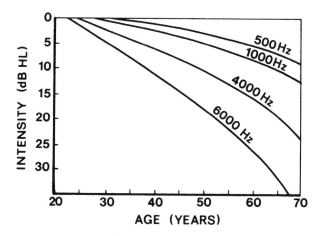

Figure 9.5.   Hearing as a function of age.

30 dB at age 65. Similar but smaller effects can be seen in the lower frequencies.

## PSYCHOLOGICAL FACTORS

A variety of "within-the-subject" factors influence the auditory threshold. The subject's motivation can have a measurable effect; it is not hard to imagine that a reward of $10 for each correct answer might have a positive effect on performance. Practice has been shown to have an important effect initially, but becomes inconsequential as the subject becomes more experienced. The listener's attention is also a critical variable. A less tangible but important factor is the internal criterion a subject sets for saying the stimulus is present or absent. Some subjects set a very liberal criterion for responding positively and will rarely miss responding to a stimulus; these subjects are likely to say they hear a tone when none is present (a false positive). The chance of a false positive occurring is reduced if the subject adopts a strict response criterion, but the number of missed stimuli will be increased in this situation. The instructions provided by the tester play an important role in the criterion chosen by the subject, and are of major concern in audiological testing.

## OTHER FACTORS

We have by no means exhausted all the factors that may influence the minimal audible signal. For example, the presence of environmental noise might partially or completely mask out the test stimulus. Physiological noise, such as blood rushing in the ear or the action of the middle ear muscles, must also be considered. Furthermore, a wide variety of pathological conditions can affect the auditory threshold, on a temporary or permanent basis.

## NORMAL HEARING AND THE AUDIOGRAM

The definition of hearing loss is very much dependent on reaching a satisfactory definition of "normal hearing." Normal hearing is usually described in the form of a graph called an *audiogram*. On the audiogram the auditory threshold is normally measured and plotted for each octave point between 250 and 8000 Hz (250, 500, 1000, 2000, 4000, and 8000 Hz). In 1969, the American National Standards Institute (ANSI) adopted standards for normal hearing levels based on the data collected by the International Standards Organization (ISO), which were released in 1964. This extensive study evaluated the hearing of a large number of otologically normal young adults who were tested in five different countries under carefully controlled conditions. The ANSI values, which are listed in Table 9.1, represent the guidelines that we accept for normal human hearing for clinical purposes.

It must be remembered that the ANSI standards represent an average value, and individual normal hearing thresholds will be scattered around this mean. Furthermore, since these values represent only young adults, the effects of aging that were discussed earlier must be taken into consideration when evaluating the hearing acuity of older persons.

## BEHAVIORAL THRESHOLD

Because so many variables affect the absolute threshold for intensity, it is most difficult to translate this important concept into a stable measurement. In order to minimize this problem, threshold is defined for clinical purposes as the minimal intensity that can be heard half (50%) of the time; this is sometimes referred to as the behavioral threshold. If one is using this operational definition, it should be remembered that a subject will occasionally perceive a tone that is below his or her behavioral threshold; this, however, will occur in less than half the presentations of this stimulus.

## HEARING LEVEL SCALE

Although it is possible to plot an audiogram in decibels of sound pressure level (re: 0.0002 dyne/cm$^2$), there are some disadvantages associated with this method. First, since normal hearing sensitivity varies from frequency to frequency, the ANSI value for mean normal threshold is different for each frequency. If you were told that a person's threshold was 25 dB SPL, this would be inadequate information because this represents normal sensitivity at 250 Hz, but 18 dB worse than normal hearing for 1000 Hz (see Table 9.1). In order to evaluate a particular threshold in terms of normality, one must know the frequency of the stimulus and have complete ANSI values available.

As Figure 9.1 shows, when normal hearing is plotted with an SPL reference, the result is a curved function. Deviations from this curved function, especially minor ones, are not easily recognized. Deviations from normality could more easily be observed if normal hearing were represented as a straight line, and all normal values were set to a zero baseline level.

Table 9.1.   Normal hearing levels[1]

| Frequency (Hz) | 125 | 250 | 500 | 1000 | 2000 | 4000 | 8000 |
|---|---|---|---|---|---|---|---|
| Intensity (dB SPL) | 45.0 | 24.5 | 11.5 | 7.0 | 9.0 | 9.5 | 13.0 |

[1] ANSI (1969).

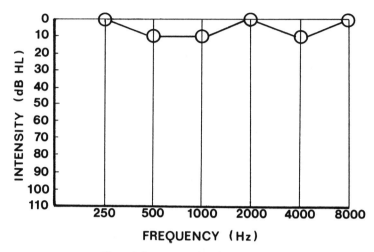

Figure 9.6.    A normal audiogram.

Remember that the decibel is a relative scale and that the base of this type of scale is arbitrarily chosen. In the SPL scale, a sound pressure (0.0002 dyne/cm²) is the zero point or base. In audiology, the hearing level (HL or HTL) scale is used for the measurement of threshold. In this scale, 0 dB always equals normal hearing threshold based on the ANSI standard. Thus, on the audiogram, 0 dB HL is normal hearing regardless of frequency. Audiometers are calibrated in dB HL so that when an audiometer is set for 0 dB HL and 1000 Hz, it automatically produces 7 dB SPL. When the audiometer is set for 0 dB HL at 250 Hz, it automatically produces 24.5 dB SPL, again the ANSI normal threshold value.

When evaluating hearing in dB HL, zero is always the normal hearing level; therefore, a person with a 50 dB (HL) threshold has a 50 dB hearing loss, whatever the frequency. In addition, normal hearing is represented, in theory, as a straight line. In reality, since normal hearing varies about the ANSI mean values, the normal audiogram may vary from a straight line. Figure 9.6 shows an audiogram of a person with normal hearing.

CONCLUSION

Audiology is the study of the measurement and rehabilitation of hearing loss. Chapter 10 discusses an alternative pathway for sound to reach the cochlea called *bone conduction*. In audiology, the most basic technique for differentiating types of hearing loss is the comparison of the normal mode of hearing, *air conduction*, to bone conduction hearing. This will be explained at the end of the next chapter.

## GLOSSARY

*absolute threshold*—The threshold of audibility. It is the point at which the minimum sound pressure level (in dB) may first be perceived.

*air conduction*—The normal route of hearing. Sound first enters the external ear canal, passes across the middle ear as vibration, and then travels to the inner ear. When an earphone is used to deliver sounds during an audiological examination, the sound is said to be delivered through "air conduction."

*ANSI*—Refers to a relatively recent standardization of the sound pressure levels that represent normal hearing for pure tones and speech. Specifically, ANSI (1969) refers to the *American National Standards Institute, Specification for Audiometers* (ANSI, S 3.6-1969).

*artificial ear*—A mechanical device on which an earphone is placed. Its purpose is to approximate the sound pressure levels produced by a sound at the tympanic membrane. An artificial ear consists of a coupler that is mechanically attached to the microphone of a sound level meter. The coupler used most frequently has a volume of 6 cc between the earphone and the microphone to approximate the volume of the average human ear canal.

*audiogram*—A graph that shows hearing loss (in dB) as a function of stimulus frequency.

*audiometry*—The method by which hearing sensitivity is measured. Pure tones and speech are the most typical signals used in audiometry.

*Bekesy audiometry*—An automated type of audiometry in which the subject tracks his own thresholds.

*binaural hearing*—Refers to hearing with two ears.

*bone conduction*—Occurs when sound passes to the inner ear through the cranial bones. During an audiological examination, a special bone conduction vibrator is used to test for bone conduction sensitivity. The usual placement is on the mastoid process.

*hearing level*—The difference (in dB) between the subject's threshold for that sound and the corresponding normal threshold. The intensity dial of an audiometer is calibrated in hearing level (in dB).

*method of adjustment*—One of the three classical psychophysical methods. In this method, the subject adjusts some aspect of the stimulus to meet some criterion set by the experimenter.

*method of constant stimuli*—One of the three classical psychophysical methods. In this method the various "constant" stimuli are presented randomly to the subject. The subject's task is to make some judgment about each stimulus presentation. For example, in an experiment dealing with the absolute threshold, the judgment for each stimulus would be "yes" or "no." That is, "Yes, I hear it," or "No, I don't hear it."

*method of limits*—One of the three classical psychophysical methods. In this method, the stimuli are adjusted by the experimenter in alternating ascending and descending series. The subject's task is to make some judgment about each of the stimuli. For example, a judgment of "yes" or "no" might be called for if one were investigating the threshold of audibility. That is, "Yes, I hear it," or "No, I don't hear it."

*minimum audible field (MAF)*—A method of measuring hearing sensitivity. It is the sound pressure level (in dB) of a tone at the threshold of audibility. It is measured in a free sound field at the place occupied by the subject's head, after the subject has been removed from the room.

*minimum audible pressure (MAP)*—A method of measuring hearing sensitivity. It is the sound pressure level (in dB) of a tone at the threshold of audibility. It is obtained using an earphone, and then measuring, or inferring, the sound pressure level at the tympanic membrane.

*monaural hearing*—Refers to hearing with one ear only.

*normal hearing*—The range of sensitivity found when a group of otologically normal individuals is tested. The individuals in the test group should not have been exposed to prolonged periods of noise. The ages of the individuals, as well as the method of threshold measurement, should be explicitly stated.

*octave*—An interval between two frequencies with a ratio of 2:1.

*presbycusis*—A general term that refers to the diminution of hearing sensitivity with advancing age.

*temporal integration*—The relationship between stimulus duration and the threshold of audibility. Within specified limits, the shorter a stimulus, the more energy will be required to reach the audible threshold.

## SUGGESTED READINGS FOR FURTHER STUDY

Green, D. M. 1976. *An Introduction to Hearing.* Lawrence Erlbaum Associates, Hillsdale, N.J.
An advanced treatment.
Harris, J. D. 1974. *Psychoacoustics*, pp. 5–15. Bobbs-Merrill Company, Inc., Indianapolis.
A brief introduction.
Richards, A. M. 1976. *Basic Experimentation in Psychoacoustics.* University Park Press, Baltimore.
A good treatment of classical methodology.

STUDY QUESTIONS

1. The minimum intensity that can be heard half of the time is called the _____.
2. The human ear is least sensitive in the _____ frequencies.
3. The upper limit of human hearing is about _____ Hz.
4. A graph of hearing thresholds as a function of frequency is known as an _____.
5. Threshold measurements that are obtained by delivering the stimuli through earphones are known as _____.
6. A modification of the psychological method called the _____ is used in audiological testing.
7. Values for normal hearing are provided by the _____ standards.
8. In the hearing level (HL) scale, 0 dB always represents _____.
9. The relationship between stimulus duration and intensity needed to reach threshold is known as _____.
10. A _____ response means that the subject has responded in the absence of a stimulus.

# CHAPTER 10
# Binaural Hearing and Bone Conduction

The patient with a severe hearing loss in one ear provides the audiologist with clinical insight into the advantages of hearing with two ears instead of one. Although very little, if any, difference is usually reported by the patient in small group conversation or in quiet situations, two problems are almost always noted:

1. The patient is often unable to judge the direction from which a sound is coming, sometimes turning in the wrong direction completely.
2. The ability to listen to and understand conversation in a noisy environment is greatly impaired. Often the background noise completely drowns out the message.

Two of the most important advantages of listening binaurally rather than monaurally are *localization* ability, and an increased capacity to separate signal from noise (selective listening). The audiologist will often recommend the use of binaural hearing aids in an attempt to restore these abilities to the bilaterally hearing-impaired patient. Despite the social stigma of wearing two hearing aids, many patients report improved functioning and great satisfaction from binaural hearing aid fittings.

## LOCALIZATION OF SOUNDS IN SPACE

For the sake of simplicity, the localization of pure tone signals in space is considered before complex signals such as speech or noise. The ear makes use of two aspects of the acoustic signal in judging its origin: the comparative time of arrival at the two ears and the comparative intensity of the signal at the two ears.

If a signal arrives either earlier or louder at one ear, it is interpreted by the central auditory system as coming from that side of the body.

### Intensity Cues for Localization

As you remember from Chapter 1, the speed of sound is constant within a medium. If the origin of a sound is neither directly in front of nor behind the head, one ear must be closer to the sound source than the other. We know that sound dissipates as it travels through a medium because of friction between the molecules. Therefore, the near ear will always get a slightly louder sound than the far ear (Figure 10.1). This small loss of intensity will occur regardless of frequency.

A second factor that affects the comparative intensity between the two ears (*interaural intensity difference* or IID) is the effect of the head itself on the sound, which is usually referred to as the *head shadow effect*.

We have already learned that low-frequency tones have long wave-lengths, whereas high frequencies have very short wavelengths (for example, the wavelength of a 1000-Hz tone is about 1.1 feet; a 100-Hz tone wavelength is about 11 feet). One of the important acoustic characteristics of tones with long wavelengths (low frequencies) is that they bend around corners easily while traveling through a medium, in opposition to short wavelengths (high frequencies) which are very directional and tend to reflect away from the head rather than bend around it (Figure 10.2).

The head shadow effect is usually greatest when the sound comes from the side of the head (90° azimuth), but is also significant when the

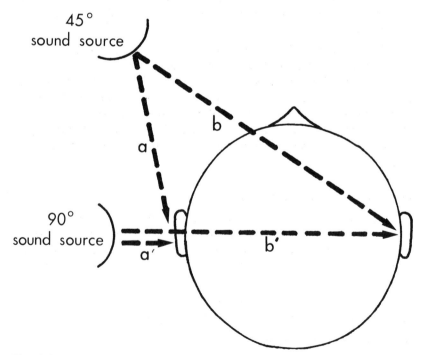

Figure 10.1. A comparison of sound reaching the near ear (a) and the far ear (b) from two different angles.

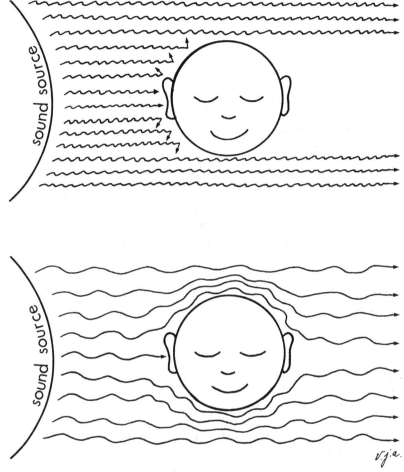

Figure 10.2.    Illustration of the head shadow effect.

sound arrives at smaller angles to the head. Figure 10.3 gives some sample values to illustrate this point.

The head shadow effect is much more important in causing an interaural intensity difference than the relatively small loss of intensity that occurs because of the distance between the near and far ear, although they are additive.

As you remember, the central auditory system interprets an interaural intensity difference as sound coming from the side getting the greater intensity. Because the head shadow occurs primarily at higher frequencies, the interaural intensity difference cue is large enough to allow the localization of tones of about 2000 Hz and higher. A similar

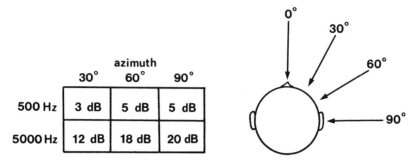

Figure 10.3.   Approximate decibel values of the head shadow effect.

phenomenon can be demonstrated and studied in the laboratory under somewhat artificial conditions. If we put earphones on a subject and present an identical pure tone to both ears, the subject will say that the tone is coming from somewhere in the middle of the head. We refer to this as *lateralization* of the tone to midline. If we increase the intensity a few decibels in either ear, the sound will clearly be lateralized to that side, confirming the interpretation of interaural intensity differences by the auditory system.

**Time Cues for Localization**

Since interaural intensity differences can only account for localization of higher frequencies, and we know that we can localize tones of all frequencies, there must be an alternative cue that accounts for localization of the lower frequencies.

We know that the speed of sound is constant within a medium, traveling at about 1100 feet per second in air regardless of frequency. If we look back to Figure 10.1, it can be seen that the distance that sound has to travel is greater to the far ear (b) than the near ear (a). Although this is true for both the 45° and 90° situations, the difference is somewhat greater for the 90° angle. Translated into time, a tone that is directed at a 45° angle to the head will arrive at the near ear approximately 0.4 milliseconds sooner than the far ear; the difference will be about 0.65 milliseconds if the azimuth is 90°.

If we go back to the laboratory situation with earphones, the literature shows that interaural differences as small as 10 microseconds (millionths of a second) have produced lateralization effects. Therefore, the much larger *interaural time differences* of up to 0.65 milliseconds are more than adequate to cue the central auditory system for the localization of low-frequency sounds.

It is interesting to note that we can actually fool the ear under certain controlled conditions. Using earphones, it is possible to trade off an interaural time difference favoring one ear with an interaural intensity difference that favors the contralateral ear. The subject's perception of the stimulus arrangement will be the middle of the head, just as it would be if the two tones were identical in all aspects.

In summary, most research supports a two-factor system in the localization of pure tones, with time cues serving the lower frequencies and intensity cues serving the higher frequencies.

**Complex Sounds**

In real life, we rarely find it necessary to localize pure tones. Most signals we are faced with are complex ones, such as noise and speech. This type of signal contains both low- and high-frequency components, and in reality both interaural intensity difference and interaural time difference are used by the auditory system when it makes localization judgments.

## HEARING IN BACKGROUND NOISE

Often the unilaterally hard-of-hearing patient finds that the difficulty he has in selective listening in a background of noise is a greater problem than the loss of localization ability. This is most often apparent in such situations as noisy restaurants or crowded parties where one tries to listen to one conversation while many others are occurring at the same time. The relative phase relationships between the two ears of the signal and noise are important in determining the detectability of the signal. By varying the phase relations, it is possible to improve intelligibility; this is known as the *binaural masking level difference* (BMLD).

To understand this, let us go back to an earphone listening situation, where precise control of the stimuli to each ear is possible.

If two tones that are identical in intensity, frequency, and phase are put into both ears, they will be perceived at midline. This bilateral stimulation with identical signals is referred to as *diotic* listening; if the signals presented to the two ears differ in any acoustic aspect (intensity, frequency, phase, etc.), the listening situation is referred to as *dichotic* listening.

If we now reverse the phase at one earphone 180° (phase opposition), keeping the intensity and frequency unchanged, the subject will now perceive the tones toward the outside of the head. The subject usually says the tone appears to be "all around the head" rather than at midline as before.

It may be easier to understand what we mean by phase in this case by looking at the movements of the tympanic membranes in these two situations. When the tympanic membranes go inward and outward together, we say that they are in phase. Conversely, when one eardrum goes in while the other goes out, the movement is out of phase. This is shown schematically in Figure 10.4.

If the signal and noise are both present binaurally, and they are perceived in the same location in space (either midline or all around the head), the intelligibility will be poor. Consider two possibilities:

A.  If the signal at both ears *and* the noise at both ears are both in phase, then intelligibility will be poor, because both signals will be perceived at midline.
B.  If the signal at both ears *and* the noise at both ears are both out of phase, then intelligibility will be poor, because both signals will be perceived "all around."

On the other hand, if we can arrange the acoustic situation so that the signal and noise are perceived in different locations, the intelligibility of the signal will be enhanced. Therefore:

C.  If the signal at both ears is in phase *and* the noise at both ears is out of phase, then intelligibility will be good because the signal is perceived at midline and the noise toward the outside of the head.

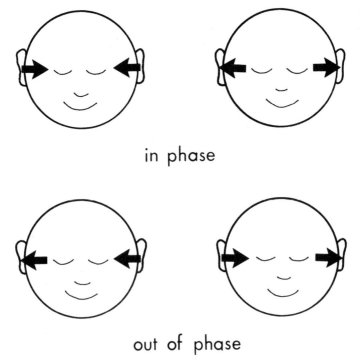

in phase

out of phase

Figure 10.4.   Relationship between eardrum movement and phase.

D.   If the signal is out of phase at both ears *and* the noise is in phase at both ears, then intelligibility will be good because the signal will be perceived toward the outside of the head and the noise at midline.

If the poorest intelligibility situations (A and B) are our baseline, then situation C will produce a 13-dB relative improvement in intelligibility of signal in noise and D will yield a 15-dB improvement. This is an example of what is meant by a binaural masking level difference. This works as well for a speech signal as for a pure tone. It is up to audiological research to devise a way for the hearing aid wearer to alter the phase relations when in a noisy environment.

**Other Binaural Effects**

Localization and increased intelligibility in noise are probably the two most important binaural effects, but a few others warrant mentioning. Hearing is about 3 dB more sensitive at threshold when one listens with two ears rather than one; this two-ear summation effect increases to a maximum of about 6 dB at 30 dB or more above threshold (*sensation level*).

There appears to be a right ear advantage for binaurally presented speech stimuli and a left ear advantage for nonspeech stimuli, like music. Although the difference may not be significant by clinical standards, it sheds some light on the functions of the two hemispheres of the brain and the relative strengths of the various pathways of the auditory central nervous system.

Many psychoacoustic abilities improve when both ears are involved. For example, the perception of loudness is greater binaurally than monaurally, and the difference limen (DL) is smaller when two ears are used.

**BONE CONDUCTION**

The normal pathway of sound is from the pinna to the cochlea through the external auditory meatus and the middle ear. This familiar route is known as *air conduction*. It is possible to apply vibration directly through the skull to the cochlea; this is known as *bone conduction*. When the sound vibration is delivered by bone conduction both cochleas are always stimulated. It seems logical therefore to discuss bone conduction as a form of binaural hearing.

When a vibrational stimulus is applied to the skull, three separate modes of bone conduction hearing occur:

1.   As the skull vibrates to and fro in response to the bone-conducted stimulus, the loosely suspended ossicular chain tends not to move

because of *inertia*. The cochlea, in essence, moves in and out relative to the stapes, causing the same effect in the organ of Corti as an air conduction signal. This is known as *inertial bone conduction*. Although it is present at all frequencies, it is thought to be of primary importance for the lower frequencies.

2.    In the lower frequencies the whole skull vibrates as a single unit. Above about 1500 Hz, the skull vibrates in a complex pattern in which the forehead may move back while the back of the skull moves forward. This causes the skull to be alternately compressed and expanded in response to the vibrations. This distortion of the skull causes fluid movement in the inner ear, leading to stimulation of the organ of Corti in a fashion that is identical to an air conduction signal. This is known as *compressional* (or distortional) bone conduction and is important for higher frequency tones.

3.    The vibration of the skull by bone conduction causes the vibration of the column of air in the external auditory meatus. These vibrations of the air column cause movement of the tympanic membrane, leading to stimulation of the cochlea through the ossicular chain. This air conduction response to a bone conduction signal is called *osseotympanic bone conduction*. This mode of bone conduction is considered to be of less importance than either the inertial or distortional modes, although bone conduction hearing results from an interaction of all three modes.

**Clinical Application of Bone Conduction**

Sound energy that strikes the skull in a sound field and is heard by bone conduction contributes little to hearing and is a relatively unimportant phenomenon. The use of a mechanical vibrator coupled to the skull to

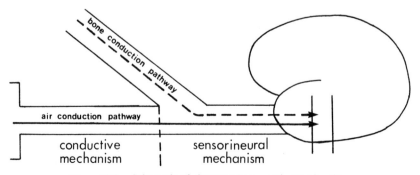

Figure 10.5.    Schematic of air versus bone conduction hearing.

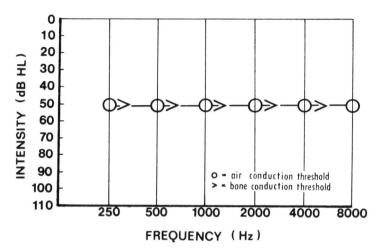

Figure 10.6.    Audiogram associated with a sensorineural hearing loss.

produce a bone conduction signal is referred to as *clinical bone conduction* and is basic to differential diagnosis in audiology.

An air conduction signal travels through the entire conductive and sensorineural mechanisms on the way to the central auditory mechanism. A bone conduction signal largely bypasses the conductive mechanism, traveling through the skull bones to the inner ear. This is illustrated in Figure 10.5.

If a patient has a sensorineural type of hearing loss, the breakdown in the hearing process will occur either in the cochlea or along the course of the VIII nerve from the cochlea to the brainstem. In the case of a conductive hearing loss, the transmission of sound will be interrupted between the pinna and the oval window.

Consider a situation in which a lesion exists somewhere in the sensorineural mechanism that causes a 50-dB hearing loss. Since both the air and bone conduction signals will be affected by the lesion in the sensorineural mechanism, the clinician will measure a 50-dB depression of hearing when testing both air and bone conduction sensitivity. Figure 10.6 shows the audiogram for this type of hearing loss.

If we move this lesion to the middle ear (for example, otosclerosis), then an air conduction signal will be affected by the lesion, but a bone conduction signal, which largely bypasses the conductive mechanism, will be unaffected. The patient will have a 50-dB loss of hearing by air conduction but no loss by bone conduction. Figure 10.7 shows the audiogram for this type of hearing loss.

Therefore, a basic rule in audiology is: If both air and bone conduction thresholds are equally depressed, the person has a sensorineural

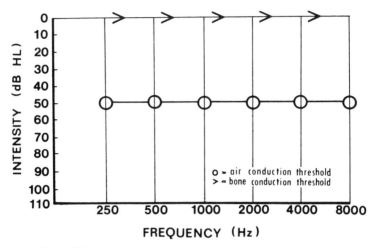

Figure 10.7.   Audiogram associated with a conductive hearing loss.

hearing loss. If air conduction hearing is depressed and bone conduction is normal, the person must have a conductive hearing loss.

## SUMMARY

Unitl this chapter, we had discussed hearing with one ear only. However, we normally listen with two ears, and with good reason. Binaural hearing allows us to localize sound and improves speech intelligibility in noise.

Bone conduction, an alternative to the normal air conduction route of sound, largely bypasses the conductive mechanism on the way to the cochlea. The comparison of air and bone conduction thresholds allows the audiologist to differentiate conductive and sensorineural hearing losses. A graph of a patient's air and bone conduction thresholds is called an audiogram.

## GLOSSARY

*binaural masking level difference (BMLD)*—Any improvement in hearing sensitivity that occurs when a signal is heard in noise, and two ears are used to listen instead of one. The BMLD is measured in decibels; it is the dB difference between the masked threshold of the signal when heard with one ear only and the masked threshold when both ears are used.

*clinical bone conduction*—A routine part of an audiometric examination. A small device known as a *bone conduction vibrator* is held against the patient's mastoid process by a metal band. Sound vibration is then delivered directly to the inner ear through the bone conduction route, and threshold is sought. The audiometric test procedure for determining bone conduction sensitivity is nearly identical to that of air conduction signals using earphones.

*compression bone conduction*—Compression bone conduction is operative at high frequencies. It is thought that the skull itself is alternatively compressed and expanded by the sound vibration. As this compression and expansion occurs, it causes the oval and round windows to expand and contract. This occurs because the cochlear fluids are incompressible. The result of this process is movement of fluid within the inner ear, which then stimulates the organ of Corti.

*dichotic listening*—A situation in which the acoustic stimuli presented to the ears differ. The sounds may differ in terms of their frequencies, intensities, phases, durations, etc.

*diotic listening*—A situation in which both ears receive identical sounds at the same instant in time.

*head shadow effect*—See *interaural intensity difference.*

*inertial bone conduction*—Operative at low frequencies; the skull is thought to vibrate as one body. The stapes, however, is not rigidly attached to the temporal bone at the oval window. When the skull vibrates, both the skull and stapes will move. However, the stapes will tend to lag behind the movement of the skull because of its resistance to movement (inertia). The result is that the stapes will move in and out of the oval window, just as in air conduction.

*interaural intensity difference*—One of the cues that facilitates auditory localization. This difference between the ears is primarily found for high-frequency tones. At these frequencies the head serves to reduce the sound reaching the ear opposite the sound source. For this reason, the term *head shadow effect* is often used to describe the phenomenon.

*interaural time difference*—One of the cues that facilitates auditory localization. The time difference between the ears arises because the ears are separated by about 11 inches, on the average. The effect of interaural time difference on localization ability is greatest for low-frequency tones.

*lateralization*—Refers to the location, within the head, of an auditory signal presented over earphones. For example, the image may appear to come from either ear, the midline, or some position between the midline and either ear.

*localization*—Refers to a situation in which a listener localizes sound in space. The listener may localize direction, or distance, or both.

*osseotympanic bone conduction*—The contribution to bone conduction hearing which occurs when the vibrating skull causes the air in the external auditory meatus to vibrate.

*sensation level* (*dB SL*)—Equal to the number of decibels that a given sound is above the threshold of audibility for a given individual.

## SUGGESTED READINGS FOR FURTHER STUDY

Green, D. M. 1976. *Introduction to Hearing*, Chapter 8. Lawrence Erlbaum Associates, Hillsdale, N.J.
Advanced and mathematical treatment of binaural hearing.
Hirsh, I. J. 1952. *The Measurement of Hearing*, Chapter 9. McGraw-Hill Book Company, New York.
A basic overview that is easy to read, but outdated.
Levitt, H., and B. Voroba. 1974. Binaural hearing. In S. E. Gerber (ed.), *Introductory Hearing Science: Physical and Psychological Concepts*. W. B. Saunders Company, Philadelphia.
Detailed discussion of binaural masking level difference.

## STUDY QUESTIONS

1. The ability to judge the source of a sound is called _____.
2. The effect of the head upon the stimulus that reaches the two ears in sound field is called the _____.
3. The normal mode of transmission of sound from the pinna to the cochlea is called _____.
4. The transmission of sound to the cochlea through the bones of the skull is called _____.
5. The localization of low-frequency stimuli depends primarily on _____ cues.
6. The localization of high-frequency stimuli depends primarily on _____ cues.
7. In a sensorineural hearing loss, air conduction _____ bone conduction.
8. The binaural phenomenon of varying phase relations between the two ears to improve intelligibility is known as _____.
9. Hearing is about _____ dB more sensitive binaurally than monaurally.
10. The _____ ear appears to have an advantage in receiving binaural speech signals.

# CHAPTER 11
# *Masking*

The familiar statement "You know I can't hear you with the water running" tells us a lot about hearing. Our ability to hear speech or other important sounds is sometimes limited by the backgrounds in which the sounds are heard. Some sounds tend to drown out or *mask* other sounds. In a more formal manner, *masking* refers to the process in which the threshold of one sound (called the signal) is raised by the simultaneous presentation of another sound (called the masker). Masking is expressed in decibels (dB). It is equal to the dB difference between the signal threshold without the masker present and the threshold with the masker present. Let's take, for example, our fictitious man who can't hear well with the water running. His initial threshold for speech without the water running might be, let's say, 20 dB SPL. The presence of the water might produce a *masked threshold* of 50 dB SPL. In other words, the water produced 30 dB of masking. Another way of saying this is that a *threshold shift* of 30 dB occurred.

Just about any kind of sound might serve as a masker or a signal. In one instance, one type of sound might serve as the signal, and in the next instance the same sound might serve as the masker. We might, for example, consider what often happens at parties or gatherings. If we try to converse with one another, the music often serves to mask the speech, making it quite difficult to understand the other person. If the same person wishes to attend to the music, the background noise of the crowd would interfere with the perception of the music. The point to be made here is that maskers and signals do not fall into exclusive categories. What serves as the signal in one case becomes a masker in another case; it all depends upon which sound is being attended to.

The hearing scientist is, of course, interested in quantifying masking phenomena because the masking process tells us about the operation of the auditory system. These phenomena can best be studied using well-controlled and easily reproducible stimuli such as pure tones, white noise, and narrow bands of noise. This chapter concentrates on the masking of pure tones, first by other tones, and then by narrow and wide bands of noise. It then looks into the relative efficiency of noise maskers and the basic mechanism that controls this efficiency. Clinical applications of masking conclude the chapter.

## MASKING OF TONES BY OTHER TONES

The masking of one tone by another provides us with important information about the nature of the masking process, and its probable relation to cochlear dynamics. Figure 11.1 is an example of pure tone masking patterns. Notice that the vertical axis represents the masking effect (in dB) produced by the various masking stimuli. The horizontal axis represents the frequencies of the masked tones. In this case the masker was a 1200-Hz tone which was adjusted to five intensity levels from 20 dB SL to 100 dB SL. Each of the five curves in the figure represents one of the masking levels.

Several important relationships are seen in Figure 11.1. The first is that for the two lowest masker levels (20 and 40 dB SL), the masking patterns are rather symmetrical around the 1200-Hz masker frequency. This simply means that the masking effects of the 1200-Hz tone on other tones in its vicinity are equally distributed above and below the frequency of the masker. Notice, however, what occurs when the level of the masker is 60 dB and above. In these cases, the patterns are asymmetrical. In other words, there are marked differences in the masking

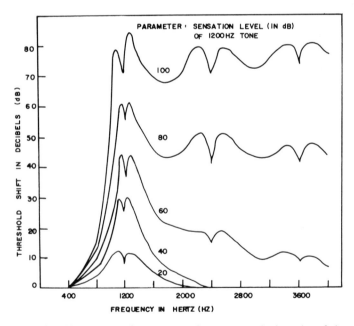

Figure 11.1.   Masking pattern of a tone on other tones as the intensity of the masker increases. (From Wegel, R. L., and C. E. Lane. 1924. The auditory masking of one pure tone by another and its probable relation to the dynamics of the inner ear. *Physics Review* 23:266–285.)

effects above and below the masker frequency. The masking effect of the 1200-Hz tone spreads rapidly upward to the higher frequencies as the masker level is increased, but extends downward in frequency to only a very limited extent. Notice, for example, that when the masker is set to 100 dB, the masking at 3600 Hz (three octaves distant from the masker) is nearly the same as at the masker frequency itself. At 400 Hz (also three octaves from the masker), however, there is no masking noted. This is usually referred to as the upward spread of masking.

The masking patterns seen in Figure 11.1 are characterized by notches in the vicinity of the masker frequency and multiples of that frequency (2400 Hz, 3600 Hz). These notches result from aural *beats* between the masker and the test signals. When the test signals are close in frequency to the masker (or multiples of the masker known as *harmonics*), fluctuations or beats in the signal levels occur, which render the signals much easier to detect. Therefore, there is less threshold shift in those frequency areas because the tones are easier to detect.

## MASKING OF TONES BY NARROW NOISE BANDS

Audible beats are eliminated from the masking process when narrow bands of noise, rather than pure tones, are used as the maskers. Figure 11.2 shows the results of a study that compared the masking effects of a 400-Hz tone and a narrow band of noise centered at nearly the same frequency. The sound pressure levels of both maskers were equal. As in the preceding figure, the vertical axis shows the masking effect in dB, while the horizontal axis shows the frequencies of the masked tones.

There are a number of relationships evident in Figure 11.2. One is that the masking pattern of the noise band is considerably smoother than the one produced by the tone. While the pure tone pattern shows the familiar notches in the region of the masker frequency and its multiples, the noise function does not. Another interesting finding is that in the region of the masker, the noise band produces considerably more masking than the pure tone masker. In fact, the difference between the two curves in the region of 400 Hz is about 20 dB. Although the noise band produces more masking in those frequencies that are more closely adjacent to the masker frequency than the tone, the masking effects of both types of sounds are about the same for the higher frequencies.

## MASKING OF TONES BY WHITE NOISE

In the two previous sections we studied the masking effects of stimuli with narrow spectra upon pure tone thresholds across the audible range.

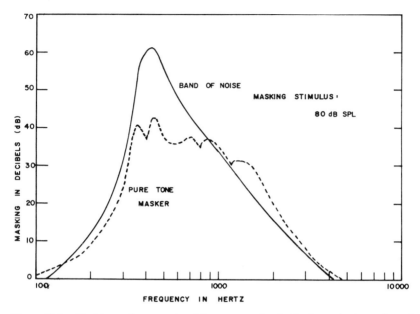

Figure 11.2.  Masking patterns produced by a narrow band of noise and a tone of equal intensity. (From Egan, J. P., and H. W. Hake. 1950. On the masking pattern of a simple auditory stimulus. *Journal of the Acoustical Society of America* 22:622–630.)

This section concentrates upon the masking effects of a frequently encountered wideband stimulus, white noise.

The results of a study of the masking effects of white noise on pure tone thresholds are presented in Figure 11.3. The vertical axis represents the masked threshold levels in dB SPL. The horizontal axis, as before, represents the frequencies of the test tones. Notice that there are four separate curves (contours) which are numbered, and another curve labeled "threshold in quiet." Each of the labeled contours shows the masked threshold levels for a different level of noise. The noise levels range from 40 dB SPL to 100 dB SPL.

What does Figure 11.3 tell us about white noise masking? The first important relationship occurs at the lower noise levels. Notice that at these lower levels the thresholds for the midfrequency tones (in the region of about 1000 Hz to 4000 Hz) are shifted to a greater extent than those frequencies above and below this region. This can be seen by the greater separation between the threshold in quiet curve and the 40-dB contour in the middle frequencies as compared with the high and low frequencies. The second important feature of the figure is that, as the level of the noise increases, the contours become flatter in appearance. This means that at higher masking intensities, the amount of threshold shift is not affected by the frequency of the stimulus. To summarize these first two relationships, then, we might say that the masked threshold levels are *dependent* upon the frequency at the lower noise levels, but are *independent* of frequency at the higher noise levels.

## MASKING AS A FUNCTION OF NOISE LEVEL

In the two previous sections we dealt with the masking effects of noise on pure tone thresholds across the hearing range. We saw that narrow bands of noise produced their greatest threshold shifts in the frequency region close to, or within, the masker boundaries. We also saw, as one might expect from its spectral composition, that white noise produced a more generalized masking pattern than the noise bands. In this section we do not look at masking patterns across frequencies, but rather examine how masking increases for a particular frequency as the noise level is raised.

The manner in which masking increases as noise level increases is the same for both narrowband and white noise maskers. The nature of this process is seen in Figure 11.4, which is a compilation of a number of studies in the area. Before we actually study the pattern of masking, it is important that we completely understand what the figure depicts. The horizontal axis shows the overall noise level of the masker in decibels.

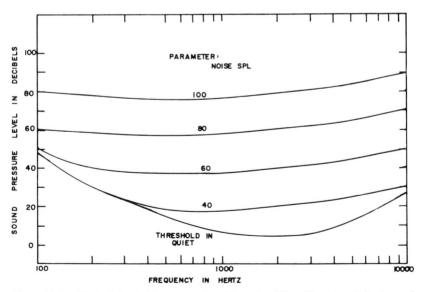

Figure 11.3.   Masked threshold contours for white noise. (From Hawkins, J. E., Jr., and S. S. Stevens. 1950. The masking of pure tones and of speech by white noise. *Journal of the Acoustical Society of America 22:*6–13.)

Notice that the level increases to the right of the figure. The masker may be either white noise or a band of noise. The vertical axis shows the threshold shift in the pure tone signal as the noise level is increased. Research has shown that the frequency of the signal may vary over a wide range (at least between 250 Hz and 8000 Hz) without any deviation from the pattern seen in the figure. If narrow bands of noise are used, the test frequency must, of course, lie at, or near, the center of the band.

The most notable feature of Figure 11.4 is that the function consists of two straight line segments which meet each other to form a kneepoint. One segment is horizontal, and remains at a 0-dB threshold shift level. The second section is diagonal. What does this tell us about the masking process? To begin with, it tells us that the intensity of the masking may be increased to a certain point without any change in the threshold of a tone. However, once the SPL of the noise reaches a critical value, there will be shifts in the threshold levels. In particular, at levels above the knee, each dB increase in the noise level will produce an equivalent shift in the threshold of the tone. In other words, above the kneepoint, there will be a 1:1 relationship between the noise level and the masking effect. The kneepoint in Figure 11.4 is frequently referred to as the *0 dB effective masking level*. It is that level of noise above which any additional noise increase will produce an equivalent threshold shift. For example, a noise that is 10 dB of effective masking will fall 10 dB above the kneepoint, and will therefore produce a 10-dB threshold shift in the tone.

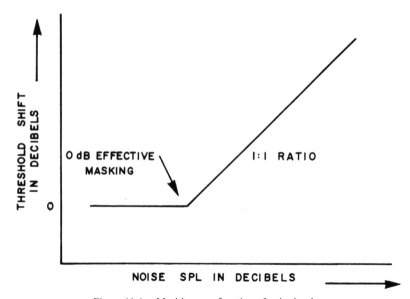

Figure 11.4.   Masking as a function of noise level.

In a similar manner, a noise that is 20 dB of effective masking will be 20 dB above the kneepoint, and produce a threshold shift of 20 dB. In summary, the effective level of the masker is equivalent to the threshold shift it produces in the test signal.

A question we might ask ourselves at this point is, "Does the noise intensity at which the knee occurs depend upon the type of noise that is used as the masker?" In other words, if we hold the frequency of the signal constant, will the kneepoint occur at the same intensity for both the narrowband noise and the white noise? For any given test frequency, the narrow band of noise will reach the 0 dB effective point (the kneepoint) at a lower intensity than the white noise. This outcome is directly related to one of the most fundamental concepts in masking: that of the *critical band*.

## THE CRITICAL BAND AND MASKING EFFICIENCY

The critical band concept in masking is based upon two main assumptions. The first is that when a tone is masked by noise, only those frequency components in the noise that lie in a narrow range around the test frequency are responsible for the masking process. Those frequency components of the noise that lie outside this "critical band" add nothing to the masking process, but only add to the loudness of the masking noise. The second assumption is that when a tone is just masked by noise, the energy content of the noise that falls within the critical band is equal to the energy of the tone.

In the preceding section, we noted that a narrow band of noise will reach the 0 dB effective masking level at a lower sound pressure level than white noise. This means that the narrowband noise is a more efficient masker than white noise because the former will induce a greater threshold shift than the latter even though both are of the same intensity (dB SPL).

The greater masking efficiency of narrowband noise than white noise is related to the spectral compositions of these maskers relative to the critical band. Narrowband noise, of course, consists of noise whose energy content is equally distributed, but restricted to a narrow frequency region. White noise consists of energy that is equally distributed over a very wide frequency range. The overall sound pressure levels of both narrowband noise and white noise are, of course, equal to the sums of the individual sound pressures for each of the component frequencies of the noises. More precisely, the sound pressure level per cycle (dB SPL/Hz) is referred to as the noise's *spectrum level*. If we were to adjust a narrow band of noise and white noise to equivalent overall SPLs, the spectrum level of the former would be considerably greater than the latter. This would occur because the overall SPL of the white noise is summed over a great many frequencies, whereas the level of the narrow band of noise is summed over a relatively narrow frequency range. Therefore, to be equivalent in their overall energy levels, the narrow band of noise would require a greater energy level per cycle than the white noise. Since the masking effect of a noise on a tone is related only to the energy that falls within the critical band, it is now readily seen why narrow bands of noise are more efficient maskers than white noise. The frequency limits of narrow bands of noise approximate the critical band. Although a white noise may have the same overall intensity as a narrow band of noise, much of the energy is not used in the masking process because it falls outside the limits of the critical band.

We learned before that the second assumption of the critical band concept is that when a tone is just masked by noise, the energy that falls within the critical band equals that of the tone. This relationship accounts for the appearance of Figure 11.4. To review for a moment, Figure 11.4 shows how masking increases as noise level increases. It consists of two line segments which meet to form a knee. One segment is horizontal, and is at a level where no masking occurs (0 dB threshold shift). The second segment is diagonal; in this latter section, masking increases in a 1:1 fashion with increased noise.

First consider what occurs in the flat section of Figure 11.4. In this section we gradually increase the noise level, but there is no masking effect. Apparently then, the noise energy that falls within the critical band is less than the threshold energy level of the tone being masked. At the kneepoint, however, the energy that falls within the critical band first equals that of the tone. This, of course, is the 0 dB effective masking point of the noise. It is also considered to be the 0 dB sensation level (SL) of the critical band. From this point on, each dB increase in the noise energy that falls within the critical band will produce an equivalent increase in the pure tone threshold. In other words, the SL of the critical band (in dB) equals the threshold shift.

To clarify the above masking process, consider Figure 11.5. If we stretch our imaginations to a considerable extent, we might consider a rain barrel to be analogous to the critical band. The barrel might be placed in a field. We might now consider the extent of the rain that falls into the barrel to be equivalent to the noise that falls into the critical band. If the rain is widespread, only a small percentage of the overall water content is collected in the barrel. If the rain is very localized, a greater percentage of the overall water level is collected. Hence, we have our equivalents of wide- and narrowband noise! One additional factor is necessary to complete the analogy—the concept of a pure tone threshold. We see in Figure 11.5 that a small rubber ball is suspended in the barrel about 1 foot above the floor. The height of the ball represents the lower

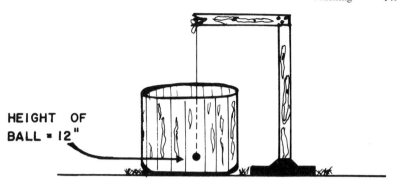

HEIGHT OF
BALL = 12"

Figure 11.5.    Illustration of the critical band concept.

threshold of the tone. Now consider what happens to the ball as the rain continues (see Figure 11.6).

When the rain (i.e., energy) first begins, the barrel (i.e., critical band) starts to fill, but the level of the ball remains constant. Thus, our threshold is unchanged. There comes a point, however, when the water level reaches the ball. This, of course, is analogous to the energy within the critical band equaling that of the tone for the first time. From this point on, each time the water in the barrel rises 1 inch, so will the height of the ball rise 1 inch.

## MASKING IN CLINICAL AUDIOLOGY

Masking, like other basic psychoacoustic phenomena, has important applications in the clinic. In the concluding section of this chapter we examine how masking is applied to routine clinical audiological practice.

The principal function of masking noise in audiometry is to eliminate the problem of *cross-hearing*. Briefly, cross-hearing is the

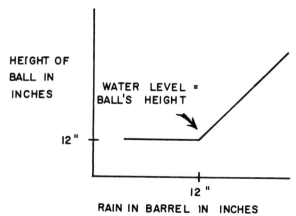

HEIGHT OF
BALL IN
INCHES

WATER LEVEL =
BALL'S HEIGHT

12"

12"

RAIN IN BARREL IN INCHES

Figure 11.6.    Height of the ball as a function of water level in the barrel.

unwanted transmission of sound from one ear to the other, which may arise under certain conditions for both air and bone conduction measurements. If cross-hearing should occur during audiometric testing, then the signal intended for one ear would actually be heard by the opposite ear. If the examiner is unaware of the possibility of cross-hearing, then he or she might erroneously report the threshold on the supposedly tested ear to be lower than it actually is.

Cross-hearing may arise in air conduction testing whenever there is a relatively large difference between the threshold levels for the two ears. This may occur in cases of unilateral impairment, where one ear is impaired, and the other normal, or when both ears are impaired, but to markedly different degrees. Conservatively speaking, the possibility of cross-hearing arises when the difference between the ears is about 40 dB or more.

Cross-hearing during bone conduction testing is a more common occurrence than during air conduction testing. Although we typically place the bone conduction vibration on the mastoid process of each ear during the audiometric examination, the sound that reaches the opposite ear may equal that on the supposedly tested ear. This is most dramatically seen when we examine an individual with profound sensorineural hearing loss on one side and normal hearing on the other. If we place the bone conduction vibrator on the impaired ear, the patient would respond to the test signals at a level that was within normal limits. This result would, of course, be due to the ability of the skull to transmit bone conduction signals from one ear to the other with little or no loss of energy. Another way of saying this is that there is no *interaural attenuation* between the ears for bone-conducted stimuli.

The problem of cross-hearing during an audiological examination is greatly reduced by introducing a masking noise into the better (or nontest) ear. This, in effect, elevates the threshold on the nontest side so that the differences in threshold sensitivity will be reduced. If masking is applied to the proper degree, then each ear will be measured in an isolated condition. Consider, for example, a case where the air conduction threshold for the right ear is 0 dB HTL, and that for the left ear is 70 dB HTL. In this case, cross-hearing might be suspected because of the rather large difference between the ears. To eliminate this possibility, we would introduce an appropriate intensity of masking noise into the better ear (right) and then test the left.

**GLOSSARY**

*clinical masking*—The process by which an ear not under test in an audiometric examination is masked to eliminate the possibility of cross-hearing.

*critical band*—A hypothetical band of frequencies that surrounds a test frequency in the masking process. When a pure tone is masked by noise, it is suggested that only those noise frequencies that fall within the critical band will be effective in the masking process. Those frequencies in the noise that lie outside the critical band will not contribute to masking. When the tone is just audible in the noise, the energy within the critical band equals that of the tone.

*cross-hearing*—The phenomenon in which the nontest ear in an audiometric examination receives the audiometric signals and the subject responds. Cross-hearing, of course, may lead to erroneous conclusions. To eliminate cross-hearing, masking noise is applied to the nontest ear.

*effective masking level*—Equal to the number of decibels that a masker shifts the threshold of the test stimulus, usually a tone. For example, a masking noise that is 15 dB effective will shift threshold 15 dB. The 0 dB effective masking point occurs at that level of the masker where a 1:1 relationship between noise level and threshold shift begins.

*interaural attenuation* (*IA*)—The insulation provided by the head between the two ears. Clinically speaking, the IA provided by the head for air-conducted sound is about 40 dB, and for bone-conducted sound is 0 dB. That is, the head provides about 40 dB of isolation between the ears for sound heard by air, and no isolation for bone-conducted stimuli.

*masked threshold*—The threshold of a sound obtained in the presence of a masker. The masked threshold is usually expressed in sound pressure level in decibels.

*masking*—Masking refers to the number of decibels that the threshold of one sound is raised by the presence of another sound.

*spectrum level*—The spectrum level of a white or narrowband noise is the sound pressure level present at each cycle of the noise. In general, if the overall sound pressure levels of white noise and narrowband noise are the same, the former would have a considerably smaller spectrum level than the latter.

*threshold shift*—The masking effect of a masker. It is measured in decibels, and it is numerically equal to the difference between the stimulus threshold in quiet, and the threshold with the masker present.

## SUGGESTED READINGS FOR FURTHER STUDY

Hirsh, I. J. 1952. *The Measurement of Hearing*, Chapter 6. McGraw-Hill Book Company, New York.
   A good introduction.

Sanders, J. W. 1978. Masking. In J. Katz (ed.), *Handbook of Clinical Audiology.* 2nd Ed. Williams & Wilkins Company, Baltimore.
Thorough treatment of applied and theoretical aspects of masking.
Studebaker, G. A. 1973. Auditory masking. In J. Jerger (ed.), *Modern Developments in Audiology.* 2nd Ed. Academic Press, New York.
A detailed examination of masking phenomena.

## STUDY QUESTIONS

1. The difference in dB of a threshold before and after the introduction of masking noise is called a _____.

2. The restricted band of frequencies around a pure tone that contributes to the masking of that tone is the _____.

3. A noise whose energy is equally distributed over a wide frequency range is _____.

4. The unwanted transmission of sound from one ear to another in audiometry is called _____.

5. The loss of energy during the transmission of sound across the head is called _____.

6. At higher intensities, the effect of a masker spreads primarily _____ in frequency.

7. A _____ noise is a more efficient masker than white noise for pure tones.

8. The intensity of the masker above which additional noise will always produce an equivalent shift is called _____.

9. The sound pressure level per cycle is referred to as the sound's _____.

10. There is no interaural attenuation between the two ears for _____ stimuli.

# CHAPTER 12
# *Loudness and Pitch*

Most people are apt to confuse the terms *loudness* and *intensity*; they think the two terms have the same meaning and are therefore interchangeable. The same thing often occurs with the terms *pitch* and *frequency*. In fact, however, each word in these pairs has a specific definition, and the pairs should not be used synonymously.

The term *loudness* represents a subjective or psychological impression that is formed within a person as a result of hearing a given sound stimulus. On the other hand, the *intensity* of a sound represents the actual physical measurement of the stimulus itself and can be measured in decibels (dB) of sound pressure (re: 0.0002 dyne/cm²) using a sound level meter. The term *pitch* refers to the psychological impression that one gains from listening to a stimulus having a given *frequency*. Thus, pitch is subjective and frequency is objective, in that one may physically measure the latter in terms of Hertz (Hz). To summarize, both loudness and pitch are subjective impressions of objective physical events, whereas intensity and frequency are the physical events themselves.

One might wonder why the differences between loudness and intensity and pitch and frequency must be so precisely defined. Should not the magnitudes of our subjective sensations correspond exactly with those intensities and frequencies of the sounds we hear? The answer is that this correspondence does not normally occur, and that the sensations of loudness and pitch grow at different rates than intensity and frequency. We saw in Chapter 2 that if one sound pressure was twice as great as another, the latter value would be 6 dB greater than the former. This occurs because doubling the sound pressure corresponds to a 6-dB increase in intensity.

If there was a one-to-one correspondence between physical intensity and subjective loudness sensation, it might be predicted that loudness sensation would double each time sound pressure doubled and be halved each time the sound pressure was halved (i.e., a 6-dB decrease). A considerable body of research has shown, however, that this is not the way the perception of loudness increases as the physical stimulus is increased. In fact, it has been demonstrated repeatedly for several types of sound that, on the average, a doubling of loudness sensation corresponds to about a threefold increase in the actual sound pressure. A 3:1 ratio between two sound pressures corresponds to about 10 dB. Thus, on the average, the sensation of loudness will double if the intensity is increased by 10 dB. Conversely, if the sound level were to be reduced by 10 dB, the loudness sensation would be halved. The above relationship is known as the "10 dB rule."

As was the case for loudness judgments, pitch is not judged by frequency alone. To illustrate this point, we could perform an experiment where two tones of different frequencies were presented to subjects. If one tone was 2000 Hz and the other 1000 Hz, would the former have twice the apparent pitch of the latter? Studies that have investigated these types of relationships have shown that the 2000-Hz tone would sound, on the average, about 1.5 times the pitch of the 1000-Hz tone. The pitch of a 4000-Hz tone would be judged as only about twice that of the 1000-Hz tone. Obviously, there is a difference between pitch and frequency.

## SCALES OF MEASUREMENT

Measurement scales are needed to measure relationships among those things we encounter each day. As we shall see, measurement scales may be loosely defined, or they may be defined with a great deal of precision. The scale may be based upon clearly observable events, or the scale may be based upon subjective impressions. For example, a very precise scale is the metric ruler, composed of millimeters and centimeters. A scale based on subjective impressions might be a scale of preference for different automobiles. This latter scale might be constructed simply by having a group of people assign numbers (i.e., scale values) to each of the automobiles in the survey. The highest number might represent the best-liked car and the lowest number the least-liked car. Those scales that seek to quantify the relationship between subjective (psychological) sensations and physical quantities are known as *psychophysical scales*. Hearing scientists have used both simple and complex scales of measurement to quantify various loudness and pitch relationships. There are four types of scales to discuss: *nominal, ordinal, interval,* and *ratio.*

### Nominal Scales

Nominal scales represent the simplest type of measurement scales. These scales are erected simply by placing the various scale items into different categories and no attempt is made to order the items. There are many areas dealing with loudness and pitch that use nominal scales of measurement. For example, these areas may involve our ability to discriminate between two stimuli. The question asked in these studies is, "What is the smallest physical difference between two stimuli that the observer can detect?" For example, if one were interested in studying loudness discrimination, various pairs of stimuli would be presented to a subject. The stimuli would vary only in their intensities, holding the frequency constant. Many different combinations would be presented. The subjects would then have to make a judgment for each pair:

1. Do the stimuli sound equally loud?
2. Do the stimuli sound different?

In this case there are two categories from which to choose, and the subject assigns one of the categories to each pair he or she listens to.

Nominal scales are not only used in discrimination tasks, but also in tasks involving the *equation of magnitudes*. The purpose of these studies is to determine those stimulus conditions where two stimuli appear to the observer to be equivalent in some respect. For example, we might be interested in knowing how intense two different frequency tones have to be to sound equally loud. As we shall see later in the chapter, this is the type of task used to establish *equal-loudness contours*. To show how this might work, we could take a 1000-Hz tone and set it to some intensity. We might then take a 2000-Hz tone and adjust its intensity so that it has the same loudness as the 1000-Hz tone. The same thing would be done with a 4000-Hz tone, a 6000-Hz tone, and so on up and down the audible spectrum. The end result would be a series of intensity values (in dB SPL) for different frequencies which all sounded equally loud to the 1000-Hz standard. A nominal scale of measurement would have been used in this experiment because the judgments fell into one of two categories—either the tones did or did not sound equally as loud as the standard tone.

**Ordinal Scales**

Ordinal scales of measurement are somewhat more complex than nominal scales because the scale items are arranged in order with respect to some common feature. Thus, these scales may be erected by procedures that require the subject to rank order the various items presented. For example, we might be interested in studying preferences for 10 ice cream flavors. We might present each of these flavors to a subject, and then ask him to rank each flavor from 1 to 10, with 10 being the most preferred flavor and 1 being the least preferred flavor. No two flavors could occupy the same rank. This scale of measurement would be ordinal because the items would be arranged in order with respect to flavor. However, using this type of scale, it would be impossible to tell about absolute differences between the items. In other words, it could not be determined whether the flavor ranked 10 was actually twice as flavorful as the flavor ranked 5, or the flavor ranked 5 was five times as flavorful as the flavor ranked 1, and so on.

Ordinal scales of loudness and pitch sensation may be erected in much the same manner as the above example. For instance, consider a study designed to rank the loudness discomfort produced by various types of aircraft as they fly over homes adjacent to an airport. Six different airplanes might be considered for the study, and these planes could be placed in rank order from 1 to 6. The rank of 6 would represent the airplane that was most uncomfortable to listen to, and the rank of 1 would represent the most comfortable airplane to listen to. As before, no two planes could share the same rank. Since the scale of measurement is ordinal, it would only be possible to determine the relative ranks among the aircraft. It would be impossible to tell from this scale whether one plane sounded twice as uncomfortable as another, or to determine any other ratio among the individual aircraft.

**Interval Scales**

Interval scales are another step removed from nominal scales in that differences between the scale items may be numerically determined. We can say, for example, that the difference between the scale numbers 10 and 15 represents the same distance as between the scale numbers 20 and 25, or 40 and 45. Consider for a moment the centigrade (or Celsius) thermometer. Using this thermometer, the difference between the interval 0°C and 10°C is equal to the difference between the interval 10°C and 20°C. Although these intervals may equal each other, and the intervals may add to each other, it is not possible to say that 20°C is twice as warm as 10°C, or that 10°C is twice as warm as 5°C or any other ratio between the temperatures. This occurs because the zero point (0°C) on the Celsius scale has been placed at an arbitrary position—at the melting point of ice.

The main point to be made here is that interval scales have the property of additivity, in addition to all the properties of nominal and ordinal scales. However, they are not absolute scales, which may tell us about ratios between the scale items. To be an absolute scale a scale should contain a "true zero" point, or that point at which the property being scaled ceases to exist. Zero degrees Celsius does not represent the absence of temperature.

Interval scales of measurement have been used to study both loudness and pitch perception. In most cases these studies have investigated what has often been termed *equal-sense distances*. The method used most often to study these equal-sense distances is the *method of bisection*. For example, if we were to study pitch perception using an interval scale we might present two different frequency tones to a subject and ask him to adjust a third variable tone so that it sounds half the pitch of the interval of the two fixed tones. This process could be continued up and down the auditory spectrum using a number of different tones as the fixed endpoints. The end result could be plotted as a scale relating equal-sense distances against frequency.

## Ratio Scales

Ratio scales of measurement contain all the properties of the previous types of scales in addition to having the property of determining exact ratios between the scale items. That is, they are capable of classification like nominal scales, ordering like ordinal scales, and determination of exact differences like interval scales. Since ratio scales have true zero points, the numbers on the ratio scale reflect actual ratios between the items. Take, for example, the common metric ruler. We know that 6 mm is twice as long as 3 mm and that 12 mm is exactly twice as long as 6 mm. In fact we can derive the exact ratio between any two scale items because there is a nonarbitrary zero point, 0 mm (0 mm is the absence of distance).

Ratio scales, then, represent the most precise scale type. The hearing scientist is particularly interested in erecting psychophysical scales that have ratio scale properties, where the scale numbers reflect the actual ratios between psychological sensations and the stimuli that produce these sensations. Several procedures have been developed to establish psychophysical scales which have ratio scale properties. These procedures generally fall into two main categories: those that ask the subject to make direct ratio judgments between two stimuli and those where the subjective magnitudes are judged directly. Let us examine in some detail how the first of these methods may be used to erect a scale of loudness.

## A Scale of Loudness

Most of the classic studies in loudness perception have used 1000-Hz tones as the stimuli. In the following example we are also concerned with the scaling of 1000-Hz tones. The reader should bear in mind, however, that the same scaling methods and principles may be extended to just about any type of auditory stimulus.

The most familiar scale of loudness is the *sone* scale. To erect a sone scale, pairs of tones are presented to each subject. The first tone in the pair is called the *standard*. The standard always assumes the same intensity level until the judgment is made. The second tone, called the *comparison*, is varied in its intensity by the subject.

Now let's look at the actual scaling procedure in some detail. To begin with, the scale must have a unit of measurement. In this case, the unit is called a *sone*. The loudness of 1 sone is arbitrarily set to be equal to the loudness of the 1000-Hz tone at 40 dB above threshold (40 dB SL). The experiment begins by presenting a stimulus pair to a subject with the 40-dB tone (1 sone) as the standard. The subject is instructed to adjust the comparison so that it sounds twice as loud as the standard. When the subject is satisfied with his or her judgment, the intensity level (in dB SL) of the comparison is noted. Since the comparison sounded twice as loud as the standard, it is assigned the loudness value of 2 sones. The 2-sone tone then serves as the standard for the next pair to be judged. Once again, the subject is asked to adjust the comparison to twice the loudness of the standard. The new intensity level of the comparison is noted after the subject is satisfied with his judgment. The loudness value of the comparison then receives the value of 4 sones, since it is twice the loudness of 2 sones. The same process continues with loudness values of 8 sones, 16 sones, 32 sones, and so forth.

Values of 1 sone or less on the scale are found in just about the same way. In this case, however, the instructions to the subjects are to adjust the loudness of the comparison tones to one-half that of the standard. For example, a loudness of 0.5 sone would sound half as loud as 1 sone. In other words, a 40-dB (1 sone) standard would be presented and the subject would adjust the comparison to one-half its loudness. The intensity level (in dB) of the comparison would then be noted and assigned the value 0.5 sone.

The results of the doubling and halving judgments, as outlined above, are a series of data points which may be graphed as shown in Figure 12.1. Figure 12.1 shows how loudness in sones is related to intensity level (reported in dB SL) of the 1000-Hz tones. To fully orient to the figure, remember that 1 sone is equivalent to 40 dB. This, of course, was our arbitrary starting point. What dB level corresponds to the loudness of 2 sones? If we draw an imaginary horizontal line from the 2-sone value on the ordinate to the graph, and then drop another line vertically to the abscissa, we see that the 2-sone value corresponds to 50 dB. In other words, we have doubled our apparent loudness (from 1 to 2 sones) by adding 10 dB. What is the dB value that corresponds to a loudness of 4 sones? If we follow the same steps as above we see that the 4-sone value corresponds to 60 dB. As before, we have doubled our loudness sensation (from 2 to 4 sones in this case) by adding another 10 dB.

By this point it may have become apparent that a relatively simple relationship exists between loudness (in sones) and intensity (in dB SL). In fact, the relationship may be graphed as a straight line (Figure 12.1). The straight line tells us that each 10-dB increase in intensity will produce, on the average, a doubling in apparent loudness. Conversely, each 10-dB decrease in intensity will be associated with an apparent halving of the loudness. This relationship has often been called the "10 dB rule."

The graph coordinates along which the sone scale is plotted in Figure 12.1 are not the type a student normally encounters. They are logarithmic rather than linear. In other words, the values that are plotted against each other are represented in a logarithmic fashion. The logarithmic nature of the ordinate (sones) is clearly evident just by looking at it. The abscissa (dB SL) may not at first glance appear to be logarithmic, but it is. Remember that decibels are logarithmic values to begin with. When a straight line graph is encountered using logarithmic coordinates (as in Figure 12.1), the graph may be referred to as a "power function." In this regard, the point to be made is that the sensation of loudness grows as a power function of intensity.

There are many sense modalities that grow as power functions. In fact, a famous experimental psychologist, S. S. Stevens, was able to postulate a general "power law" to account for many of our subjective sensations.

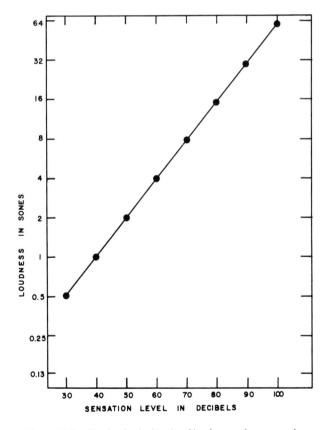

Figure 12.1.   Psychophysical scale of loudness—the sone scale.

## A Scale of Pitch

A psychophysical pitch scale might be erected using a similar method. If one were to develop such a scale there would, once again, be standard and comparison stimuli. The standards in this case would be various frequency tones set at a constant loudness level. The frequency of the comparison tones could be varied by the subject to satisfy the pitch ratio specified by the experimenter. For example, the subject might adjust the comparison to one-half the apparent pitch of the standard. To avoid biasing the experiment, the loudness levels of the comparison stimuli would always have to equal the loudness levels of the standards.

Figure 12.2 shows the most familiar scale of pitch—the *mel* scale. Just as the scale of loudness requires a basic measurement unit, the sone, the pitch scale also requires a basic unit. In this instance, the unit is called a *mel*, and 1000 mels are arbitrarily set to equal the pitch produced by a 1000-Hz tone at a sound pressure level of 40 dB. Let's look at the mel scale in detail to see how pitch is related to frequency.

The first thing to note about the mel scale is that the value of 1000 mels corresponds to 1000 Hz. This, of course, is our arbitrary measurement unit. A question we might ask is "What frequency does a pitch of 2000 mels correspond to?" In other words, what frequency sounds twice the pitch of our 1000-mel standard? If we draw a horizontal line from the

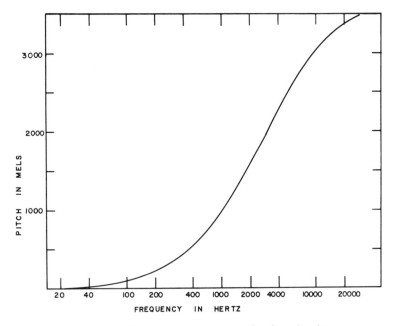

Figure 12.2.   Psychophysical scale of pitch—the mel scale.

2000-mel coordinate to intersect the scale, and then drop the line vertically to the frequency axis, we see that 2000 mels corresponds to a frequency of about 3000 Hz. The frequency must triple (from 1000 Hz to 3000 Hz) in order for the average individual to judge the pitch as double. Now take the 2000-mel (3000 Hz) standard, and see what frequency corresponds to twice its pitch (i.e., 4000 mels). We see from the scale that the 4000-mel value is not plotted because it exceeds 10,000 Hz. In other words, to double the pitch of 2000 mels requires that the frequency be raised well above 10,000 Hz. Thus, the ratio between the standard (3000 Hz) and the adjusted comparison tone would exceed a 3:1 frequency ratio for a doubling of subjective pitch. Finally, look at the value 500 mels, or one-half the pitch of the 1000-mel standard. What frequency does it correspond to? If we extend another line from the 500-mel point to the curve and then downward, we note that the frequency that is intersected is about 400 Hz. Thus, half the pitch of the 1000-Hz standard is less than one-half of that frequency.

In sum, the relation of pitch to frequency does not adhere to the "power law" as described earlier for the sense of loudness. Pitch appears to grow in a predictable, but not simple, manner.

## EQUAL LOUDNESS

Earlier in the chapter, in our discussion about various scale types, we spoke briefly about studies that equate loudnesses for different frequencies. In other words these studies determined the sound levels for various frequency tones that give the same subjective loudness impressions. If we had a representative sampling of many different frequency tones across the hearing range, all producing the same loudness sensation, we would be able to plot these data as an *equal-loudness contour*. Let us see how an experiment of this sort might be performed, and what the form of equal-loudness contours looks like.

To begin our experiment we must have some unit of measurement. This unit in this case is called a *phon*, and the number of phons is equal to the loudness produced by a 1000-Hz tone at any given intensity (in dB SPL). For example, if the 1000-Hz tone has SPL of 60 dB it would have a loudness level of 60 phons. If the 1000-Hz tone has SPL of 15 dB, it has a loudness level of 15 phons, and so on. The loudness level (in phons) of any other frequency tone is numerically equal to the SPL of the 1000-Hz tone judged to be equally loud. This may at first appear to be a bit confusing, but taking a closer look at the actual scaling process should clear matters.

As in the previous sections, two tones are presented to a subject, and a judgment is made. In this case the judgment is one of equality: "Do the tones sound equally loud, or do they not sound equally loud?" The reader might have guessed that the 1000-Hz tones serve as the standard stimuli and assume a given phon level. The comparison stimuli are various frequency tones across the hearing range, which can be varied in intensity to match the loudness of the standards.

Figure 12.3 shows the form of equal loudness contours. The numbers shown on each of the contours represent a given phon value. For example, the 60-phon contour represents the loudness matches between the 1000-Hz standard tone (at SPL of 60 dB) and other frequency tones which are adjusted in loudness to match that standard. In the same way, the 40-phon contour presents the loudness matches between the 1000-Hz standard, at SPL of 40 dB, and many other tones.

The most apparent feature of the contours is that they seem to flatten out as the intensity of the standard is increased. Stated another way, this means that the effect of frequency on loudness is present to a greater extent when the sound level is low than when the sound level is high. To illustrate this relationship, look at the 20- and 120-phon contours in some detail. Notice that a 100-Hz tone must be raised to about 40 dB to produce a loudness level of 20 phons, and to 125 dB to have a loudness level of 120 phons. In the first instance, the 100-Hz tone had to be raised 20 dB higher than the standard to sound equally loud. In

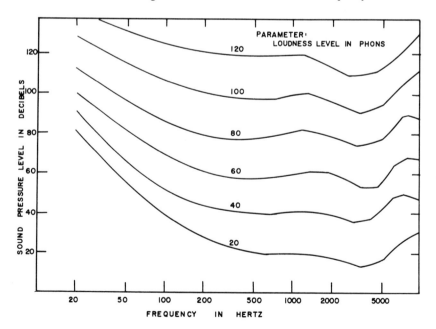

Figure 12.3.    Equal-loudness contours. (From Robinson, D. W., and R. S. Dadson. 1956. *British Journal of Applied Physics 7:* 166–181.)

the second instance, the 100-Hz tone only had to be 5 dB higher than the standard to sound equally loud.

## ABNORMAL LOUDNESS PERCEPTION

Until now we have dealt with the normal ear and how it responds as intensity is increased above threshold. The normal perception of loudness is altered considerably in persons with a cochlear hearing loss because of a disorder called *recruitment*. Recruitment is an abnormally rapid increase in perceived loudness as the stimulus intensity is raised above threshold. In other words, a given increase in intensity produces a disproportionately large increase in the loudness perceived by the patient.

Since recruitment accompanies most cochlear hearing losses and is not present in retrocochlear, central, or conductive hearing losses, the audiologist can use the presence or absence of recruitment to assist in differential diagnosis. Demonstrating the presence of recruitment would be indicative of cochlear pathology.

The most familiar method used in the clinic to determine the presence of recruitment is called the *alternate binaural loudness balance test* (ABLB). This test is usually done when the patient has one normal and one impaired ear. The audiologist compares the growth of loudness in the two ears by alternately presenting a tone to each ear. We know that a normal ear should not have recruitment. If both the normal ear and the abnormal ear perceive tones of equal *sensation level* (SL, the number of decibels above the individual's threshold) as equally loud, then the abnormal ear also cannot have recruitment. In other words, if a 50-dB SL tone in the normal ear sounds as loud as a 50-dB SL tone in the impaired ear, the ears must be perceiving loudness equally. Therefore, the impaired ear is not displaying recruitment. However, if 50 dB SL in the normal ear sounds as loud as a lesser intensity (say 30 dB SL) in the impaired ear, we know that recruitment is present because the impaired ear is perceiving loudness abnormally. This finding would suggest the presence of a lesion of cochlear origin.

The measurement of recruitment is an important part of the differential testing procedure in audiology known as the site of lesion battery. The ABLB is only one test of several that utilizes loudness perception to evaluate hearing loss. Another test, the SISI, is discussed in the next chapter.

## GLOSSARY

*alternate binaural loudness balance (ABLB) test*—A clinical procedure by which the phenomenon of loudness recruitment is demonstrated.

*equal-loudness contour*—A curve that relates equal loudness sensation (in dB SPL) for various frequency sounds. The reference frequency against which the loudness of all other frequencies is compared is 1000 Hz. (See *phon*.)

*loudness*—The aspect of sound perception in which sounds may be ordered from "soft" to "loud." Loudness perception is principally related to stimulus intensity, but frequency also plays a role.

*loudness recruitment*—A phenomenon very often associated with cochlear hearing loss. When this occurs, loudness sensation increases more rapidly than normal at levels just above threshold. However, at higher levels the sensation of loudness becomes normal.

*mel scale*—A psychophysical scale of pitch perception. The unit of the mel scale is the *mel*. One thousand mels are equivalent to a 1000-Hz tone set at a sound pressure level of 40 dB.

*phon*—A unit of loudness. The number of phons for any frequency tone is equal to the sound pressure level (in dB) of a 1000-Hz tone judged to be equally loud. (See *equal-loudness contours*.)

*pitch*—The psychological perception of frequency. It is that aspect of a sound which can be ordered from "high" to "low." Pitch is primarily related to frequency in such a way that low frequency sounds produce low pitches, and high frequencies sounds produce high pitches.

*power function*—A straight line function when two variables are plotted on log-log coordinates.

*power law*—Mathematically describes the way in which many sensations grow as stimulus intensity is increased. In general, the law states that many senses grow as a *power function* of intensity. This means that equal stimulus ratios will always produce equal ratios of sensation. (See *power function*.)

*psychophysical scale*—A function that relates subjective perceptions to physical events. That is, these scales seek to quantify the relationships between physical and psychological events. Both the sone and mel scales are examples of psychophysical scales.

*ratio production*—A psychophysical scaling method in which the subject is required to produce a prescribed ratio between two stimuli. The ratios most often set by the subjects are either 2:1 or 1:2.

*scales of measurement*—There are four levels of precision in measurement. These apply to physical as well as psychological events. From the lower to the higher levels, there are the nominal, ordinal, interval, and ratio scales. These scales are distinguished from each other by several criteria. In general, the lower level scales require little mathematics, and only classification is considered. The higher level scales are more amenable to mathematical and statistical operations.

*sone*—An arbitrary unit of loudness. It is defined as the loudness of a 1000-Hz tone set at 40 dB above threshold (40 dB sensation level).

*sone scale*—A ratio scale of loudness in which the arbitrary unit of loudness is the sone.

*standard stimulus*—In many psychophysical experiments two signals are presented to the subject for comparison. The first is usually the *standard* and the second, the *comparison*. The subject is then asked to make some judgment of the comparison relative to the standard. For example, the subject may be asked to judge the loudness of the comparison relative to the standard.

## SUGGESTED READINGS FOR FURTHER STUDY

Licklider, J. C. R. 1951. Basic correlates of the auditory stimulus. In S. S. Stevens (ed.), *Handbook of Experimental Psychology*. John Wiley & Sons, New York. Classic detailed treatment.

Richards, A. M. 1976. *Basic Experimentation in Psychoacoustics*, Chapter 4. University Park Press, Baltimore. A basic experimental approach to the assessment of loudness.

Stevens, S. S. 1959. The psychophysics of sensory function. In W. A. Rosenblith (ed.), *Sensory Communication*. MIT Press, Cambridge, Mass. A well-written, complete discussion.

STUDY QUESTIONS

1. The psychological impression related to intensity is known as _____.

2. Pitch is the psychological correlate of _____.

3. A _____ scale is the most precise scale for measurement.

4. In order to produce a doubling of perceived loudness, about _____ dB must be added to the stimulus.

5. The _____ states that equal intensity ratios produce equal loudness ratios.

6. The arbitrary unit of loudness equal to a 1000-Hz tone of 40 dB SPL is known as a _____.

7. An abnormally large increase in perceived loudness above an impaired threshold is known as _____.

8. A scale that quantifies the relationship between subjective sensation and physical quantities is known as a _____ scale.

9. A clinical test of loudness recruitment that uses both ears is called the _____.

10. The unit of pitch is the _____.

# CHAPTER 13
# Differential Sensitivity

In Chapter 9 we studied absolute thresholds, or the lower limits of our auditory awareness. At that time we defined an absolute threshold as the smallest intensity that could be perceived by a listener half (50%) of the time. We are also concerned with other types of auditory thresholds that occur well above the lower limits of hearing. Foremost among these are *difference limens* (*DL*), or differential thresholds, which measure the smallest differences between two stimuli that can first be perceived by a listener. Operationally speaking, difference limens are often defined as the smallest stimulus differences perceived half of the time.

Difference limens may be expressed in absolute or relative terms. What this means simply is that the minimum stimulus separation just perceived as noticeably different may be reported in the actual physical units themselves, or the separation may be divided by the original stimulus value to form a fraction. Let's make up an experiment that will illustrate the DL. In this experiment we have a weight of 90 grams, which we will call the standard. Additional weight can be added to the standard in 1-gram steps. The experimental problem in this instance would be to determine the difference limen for weight, or $DL_{wt}$. In other words, we seek to find the number of additional grams necessary to make a judgment of just noticeably heavier. For example, suppose that the overall weight had to be increased to 93 grams to be first noticed as heavier by the subject of our experiment. If we specified this DL in absolute terms, then the value would be 3 grams, or the difference between the standard and the final weight (comparison). If the DL were reported in relative terms, then the value would be $\frac{3}{90}$ or 0.03. In this case, the absolute change was divided by the standard.

## WEBER'S LAW

A fundamental question we might ask about our discrimination abilities is whether or not there is regularity in the size of the DL across the stimulus range for any given sense modality. In other words, does a consistent relationship exist between the standard stimuli and the increment judged to be just noticeably different? Two types of relationships are possible. First, we might suppose that the absolute increment always equals the same stimulus value across the entire stimulus range. Second, there may be a constant proportion between the absolute increment and the individual standard stimuli. Research has shown that the notion of a constant absolute increment is not supported. On the other hand, the notion of a constant proportion has considerable support in the literature, but there are some notable qualifications.

The fraction obtained when the absolute increment is divided by the standard is known as the *Weber fraction* or *Weber ratio*. It derives its name from the work of Ernst Weber who, in 1834, proposed that in order for one stimulus to be judged as just noticeably different from another, the second always had to be increased by a constant proportion of the first. Another way of saying this is that a stimulus must be increased by a constant proportion of itself to be judged just different. This relationship is known as *Weber's law*. More formally, Weber's law may be written as:

$$\frac{\Delta I}{I} = K$$

where the term $\Delta I$ (delta $I$) represents the absolute change in the stimulus necessary to produce a judgment of just noticeably different, $I$ represents the standard stimulus, and $K$ represents the constant.

The nature of Weber's law can be examined in more detail by using the lifted weight experiment once again. In our experiment there will be three standard weights: 30, 60, and 90 grams. The purpose of the experiment is to determine how much additional weight must be added to each of the three standards to be judged as just heavier. If Weber's law were to hold true, then we would expect that the weight increments would always be a constant fraction of the standards. It is known that the *Weber constant* in the case of lifted weights is about one-thirtieth ($\frac{1}{30}$). Therefore, our subjects will need an increase of $\frac{1}{30}$ of the standard weight to judge a just noticeably heavier difference. In the present case, we should find that $\Delta W$ would equal 1, 2, and 3 for the 30-, and 60-, and 90-gram standards, in that order. Thus, the 30-gram standard would have to be increased to 31 grams, the 60-gram standard would have to be increased to 62 grams, and the 90-gram standard would have to be increased to 93 grams to be judged as just noticeably heavier.

A considerable effort has been spent in determining the universality of Weber's law across many sense modalities. Weber's law would, of course, predict that the constant $(K)$ would remain unchanged for all intensity levels within one sense modality, but that the value of the constant might change from one sense to another. In general, it has been found that the Weber fraction does remain fairly stable for many senses, but only in the middle intensity ranges. At the lower and upper extremes of the intensity ranges, the Weber fractions tend to increase. In other words, our discrimination abilities are generally better in the mid-ranges than at the extremes.

## HEARING DIFFERENCE LIMENS

There are many facets of hearing that require us to discriminate between or among small, but very important, sound changes. Without this fine discrimination ability, our understanding of speech, as well as the perception of other important auditory signals, would be severely limited. In this section we discuss three important aspects of our differential sensitivity to sound: intensity, frequency, and temporal (time) discrimination.

### Intensity Discrimination

The difference limen for intensity $(DL_I)$ is generally measured by presenting two tones of the same frequency to the listeners. The first tone, the standard, remains fixed at some intensity level. The second tone, the comparison, varies in small dB steps around the standard. The listening task is to determine when the tones are just noticeably different in their loudness sensations.

Figure 13.1 shows the DL for intensity for 1000-, 4000-, and 10,000-Hz stimuli. Notice that the DLs are measured in both absolute ($\Delta I$ in dB) and relative ($\Delta I/I$) terms. The absolute values are listed on the left side and the relative values (the Weber fractions) are listed on the right-hand side. The horizontal axis shows the sensation levels (in dB) of the standard tones. There are three separate curves shown, one for each of the test frequencies (1000, 4000, and 10,000 Hz).

What does Figure 13.1 tell us about our ability to discriminate intensity differences? The first overall impression that we gain is that all three test frequencies show similar patterns, although there are differences in the actual DL values. Each plot slopes downward as the sensation levels (loudness) of the tones are increased to about 40 to 50 dB. Thereafter, the DL values remain relatively stable. This tells us that at low sensation levels (soft sounds) we are less sensitive to sound intensity changes than at higher sensation levels. Once the sound intensity reaches about 40 to 50 dB SL, however, our intensity discrimination abilities are most acute, and they remain at this level of acuity as loudness increases to high levels.

Figure 13.1 also shows us that our ability to discriminate intensity is affected by the frequency of the tones. At lower sensation levels, the

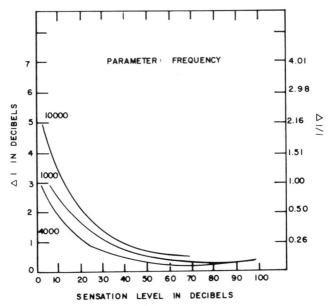

Figure 13.1.    Difference limen for intensity in absolute and relative terms. (From Reisz, R. R. 1928. Differential intensity sensitivity of the ear for pure tones. *Physics Review* *31*:867–875.)

10,000-Hz tones are considerably more difficult to discriminate between than the 1000-Hz and 4000-Hz tones; however, these differences decrease as the sensation level of the tones increases.

We noted before that Weber's law held for many sense modalities in the middle intensity ranges. This appears to be the case for intensity discrimination since the Weber fractions remained essentially stable above 40 to 50 dB SL. On the other hand, Weber's law clearly does not hold at the lower sensation levels for intensity discrimination.

### Frequency Discrimination

The difference limen for frequency ($DL_F$) is determined by presenting two tones to the listeners. The first tone, the standard, remains fixed at one frequency at all times. The second tone, the comparison, varies in small frequency steps around the standard. The listening task in this case is to determine when the tones are just noticeably different in their pitch sensations.

Two important questions come to mind with reference to DL for frequency. The first is, "For any given frequency, does the $DL_F$ change as the loudness level changes?" The second question is, "For any given loudness level, does the $DL_F$ change with frequency?"

Figure 13.2 shows how the DL for frequency (in relative terms, $\Delta F/F$) changes for various frequency tones as loudness level is increased. Although the absolute sizes of the DLs vary from frequency to frequency, all of the curves show similar patterns. In general, each curve slopes rapidly downward as the loudness level is increased to about 20 phons, and then the functions start to level off.

What does Figure 13.2 tell us about our frequency discrimination abilities for various frequency tones? We are relatively insensitive to frequency changes at low loudness levels, but as the loudness level is increased, our discrimination abilities improve. We are most sensitive to frequency changes when the loudness levels are about 30 phons and higher. Although the above relationships hold true for each of the frequencies tested (250 Hz to 4000 Hz), Figure 13.2 shows that our overall sensitivity to some frequencies is better than others. Remember that the lower the Weber fraction, the better the frequency discrimination ability.

Our discussion of the difference limen for frequency to this point has

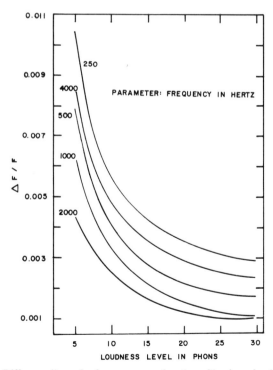

Figure 13.2. Difference limen for frequency as a function of loudness level. (From Harris, J. D. 1952. Pitch discrimination. *Journal of the Acoustical Society of America* 24:750–755.)

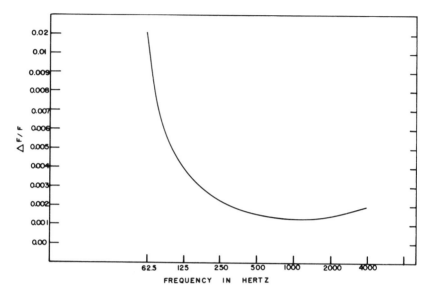

Figure 13.3.    Difference limen for frequency as a function of frequency. (From Harris, J. D. 1952. Pitch discrimination. *Journal of the Acoustical Society of America 24*:750–755.)

dealt with the effect of loudness on sensitivity. The other question that was posed dealt with the effect of frequency on sensitivity. We just saw, in a very general way, that our overall sensitivity was better at some frequencies than at others. Now let us look at this particular relationship in greater detail.

Figure 13.3 shows the relative difference limen ($\Delta F/F$) as a function of frequency. The figure clearly shows that $DL_F$ decreases rapidly as the frequency is raised to 125 Hz, but thereafter remains fairly constant. Although the DL values remain relatively unchanged from 500 Hz to 4000 Hz, our best sensitivity appears to lie in the 1000-Hz to 2000-Hz frequency region. Once again, Weber's law appears to hold for the middle values in the range, but not at the lower extremes.

**Time Discrimination**

The difference limen for time ($DL_T$) may be measured in a similar manner to intensity and frequency. Generally, two signals are presented in succession. The first signal, the standard, has a fixed duration, and remains at a given loudness level. The second signal, the comparison, varies in small duration steps around the standard. The loudness level of the comparison equals that of the standard. The subject's task in this case is to determine when the signals are just noticeably different in their apparent lengths.

Figure 13.4 shows how the relative difference limen for time ($\Delta T/T$) varies as the duration of the standard signal is lengthened. The effect is quite clear. As the duration of the standard increases from 0.4 milliseconds (0.0004 seconds) to 4.0 milliseconds (0.004 seconds), there is a rapid decline in the Weber fractions. When the standard varies from 4.0 milliseconds to 400 milliseconds (0.4 seconds), the decrease continues, but at a considerably slower pace than before. Other studies in this area have shown this trend to continue to at least 1000 milliseconds (1 second).

In sum, we may conclude that our sensitivity to time differences improves as the length of the stimulus increases.

### Clinical Use of the Difference Limen

Many of the tests that we use routinely in the audiology clinic are based upon well-established normal hearing phenomena which are, in one way or another, altered by various types of auditory disorders. The differential sensitivity to various aspects of sound falls into this category. A considerable effort has been made in developing clinical tests based upon DLs, or closely related discrimination abilities.

Perhaps the most thoroughly investigated aspect of differential sensitivity is the difference limen for intensity ($DL_I$). This is because

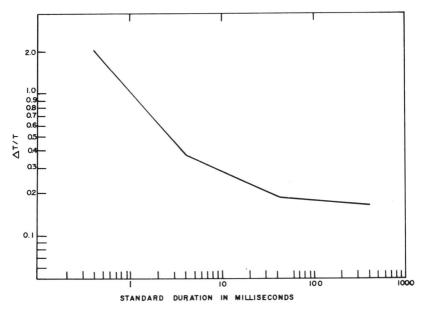

Figure 13.4.    Difference limen for time. (From Small, A. M., and R. A. Campbell. 1962. Temporal differential sensitivity for auditory stimuli. *American Journal of Psychology* 75:401–410.)

listeners with cochlear disorders generally produce smaller $DL_I$s near threshold (i.e., at low sensation levels) than their normal-hearing counterparts.

Figure 13.5 shows the absolute $DL_I$ (in dB) as a function of sensation level for normal ears and for ears with cochlear damage. The normal function should be familiar to us by now (see Figure 13.1). It shows that our sensitivity to intensity changes tends to be relatively poor at very low sensation levels, but improves rapidly as the sensation level is increased. Notice that the curve for the cochlear-impaired ears takes a markedly different shape than the normal ears. What we see here is that the $DL_I$s remain relatively constant as the sensation level is increased. In other words, the impaired ears are considerably more sensitive to intensity changes at low sensation levels than normal ears. As the stimulus level is increased, however, this detection advantage disappears.

The fact that ears with cochlear damage show reduced $DL_I$s (increased sensitivity) at low sensation levels has inspired a number of clinical procedures in the past. Some of these procedures actually measured the $DL_I$ at various sensation levels, while other procedures compared the differences in $DL_I$ values between relatively low sensation levels and higher sensation levels. The most well-known contemporary clinical procedure based upon $DL_I$ is the *short increment sensitivity index* (better known as the *SISI test*). This test does not actually

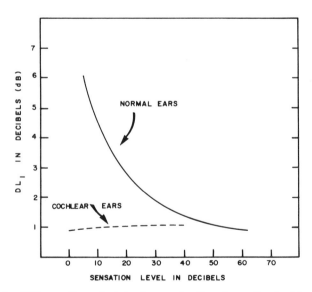

Figure 13.5.   Difference limen for intensity as a function of sensation level in normal and cochlear-impaired ears. (Adapted from Denes, P., and R. E. Naunton. 1950. The clinical detection of auditory recruitment. *Journal of Laryngology 64:*375–398.)

measure the $DL_I$, but rather it makes use of the fact that an ear with cochlear damage has a smaller DL at low sensation levels than a normal ear. A steady pure tone is presented at 20 dB SL. Superimposed upon this tone are a series of 1-dB intensity increments. These increments last for 200 msec and occur every 5 sec. The patient signals whenever he hears the small increase in loudness produced by the 1-dB increments. In general, ears with cochlear damage will produce high SISI scores since they will be able to perceive the 1-dB increments at the low sensation level used during the test. Normal ears are unable to detect these small increments at low sensation levels and, therefore, the SISI scores for these ears will be low. In this way, the DL can be used to differentiate normal ears from ears with cochlear damage.

### GLOSSARY

*absolute difference limen*—The least stimulus increment (or decrement) necessary to judge one stimulus as just noticeably different from another. The absolute DL may be expressed as $\Delta I$ in dB, $\Delta F$ in Hz, $\Delta t$ in milliseconds, or any other stimulus value under investigation.

*difference limen* $(DL)$—The smallest increment (or decrement) in a stimulus value that is first perceived. By convention, the DL is considered to be a statistical value. It is generally taken to be the stimulus value that elicits a response of just noticeably different one-half (50%) of the time. Difference limens may be found for many aspects of auditory experience.

*frequency discrimination* $(DL_F)$—The least frequency separation between two tones perceived as just noticeably different. The $DL_F$ may be expressed in absolute terms ($\Delta F$ in Hz), or in relative terms, where the absolute increment ($\Delta F$) is divided by the original frequency ($F$).

*intensity discrimination* $(DL_I)$—The least intensive difference between two stimuli perceived as just noticeably different. The $DL_I$ may be expressed in absolute terms ($\Delta I$ in dB), or in relative terms, where the absolute increment ($\Delta I$) is divided by the original stimulus ($I$).

*relative difference limen*—The fraction formed when the absolute change required for one stimulus to be judged as just noticeably different from another is divided by the original stimulus value. Mathematically, the relative DL takes the form $\Delta I/I$ for intensity.

*time discrimination*—The smallest difference in stimulus durations between two stimuli judged as just noticeably different. The $DL_T$ may be expressed in absolute terms (milliseconds), or in relative terms, where the absolute time increment ($\Delta_T$) is divided by the original stimulus length (T).

*Weber fraction*—The fraction obtained when the absolute stimulus increment for a judgment of just noticeably different is divided by the original stimulus value. For example, if the difference limen for frequency ($DL_F$) were under investigation, the form of the Weber fraction would be $\Delta F/F$, where $\Delta F$ was the absolute increment in frequency noticed as just different and $F$ was the original frequency.

## SUGGESTED READINGS FOR FURTHER STUDY

Hirsh, I. J. 1952. *The Measurement of Hearing*, Chapter 7. McGraw-Hill Book Company, New York.
An excellent overview.
Littler, T. S. 1965. *The Physics of the Ear*, Chapter 7. Pergamon Press, Oxford.
A more advanced treatment.

**STUDY QUESTIONS**

1. The smallest difference that can be perceived between two stimuli is known as the _____.
2. _____ states that a stimulus must be increased by a constant proportion of itself to be judged as just noticeably different.
3. The Weber fraction remains stable for many senses in the _____ of the intensity range.
4. The lower the Weber fraction, the _____ the discrimination ability.
5. A clinical test for cochlear pathology, based upon differential sensitivity, is the _____.

# ANSWERS TO STUDY QUESTIONS

## ANSWERS TO CHAPTER 1

1. Hz
2. frequency
3. amplitude
4. period
5. simple harmonic motion

6. complete cancellation
7. decrease
8. sine wave
9. fundamental frequency
10. complex tone

## ANSWERS TO CHAPTER 2

1. 0.0002 dynes/cm²
2. intensity
3. pressure
4. linear
5. absolute

6. 6
7. 0
8. 140
9. 6
10. logarithm

## ANSWERS TO CHAPTER 3

1. cochlea
2. conductive
3. external auditory meatus
4. central hearing loss
5. VIII

## ANSWERS TO CHAPTER 4

1. outer ear
2. otoscope
3. pars flaccida, pars tensa
4. radial, circular
5. stapes

6. malleus
7. Eustachian tube
8. stapedius, tensor tympani
9. promontory
10. attic

## ANSWERS TO CHAPTER 5

1. impedance
2. mass, stiffness, friction
3. condensation effect
4. lever action
5. atresia

6. 30 dB
7. otosclerosis
8. myringotomy
9. serous otitis media
10. tympanoplasty

## ANSWERS TO CHAPTER 6

1. modiolus
2. cochlea, vestibule, semicircular canals
3. endolymph
4. cochlear, vestibular
5. otolith system, semicircular canals

6. scala vestibuli, scala tympani, scala media
7. organ of Corti
8. hair cells
9. round window
10. temporal

## ANSWERS TO CHAPTER 7

1. sensorineural
2. organ of Corti
3. traveling wave
4. basal
5. place

6. cochlear microphonic
7. presbycusis
8. retrocochlear
9. rubella
10. Ménière's disease

## ANSWERS TO CHAPTER 8

1. synapse
2. medulla
3. afferent
4. decussation
5. temporal

6. cerebellopontine
7. superior olivary complex
8. auditory agnosia
9. cochlear nucleus
10. auditory radiations

## ANSWERS TO CHAPTER 9

1. behavioral threshold
2. low
3. 23,000
4. audiogram
5. MAP

6. method of limits
7. ANSI
8. normal hearing
9. temporal integration
10. false positive

## ANSWERS TO CHAPTER 10

1. localization
2. head shadow effect
3. air conduction
4. bone conduction
5. interaural time difference

6. interaural intensity difference
7. equals
8. binaural masking level difference
9. 3–6
10. right

## ANSWERS TO CHAPTER 11

1. threshold shift
2. critical band
3. white noise
4. cross-hearing
5. interaural attenuation

6. upward
7. narrowband
8. 0 dB effective masking
9. spectrum level
10. bone conduction

## ANSWERS TO CHAPTER 12

1. loudness
2. frequency
3. ratio
4. 10
5. power law

6. sone
7. recruitment
8. psychophysical
9. ABLB
10. mel

## ANSWERS TO CHAPTER 13

1. difference limen
2. Weber's law
3. middle
4. better
5. SISI test

# Index